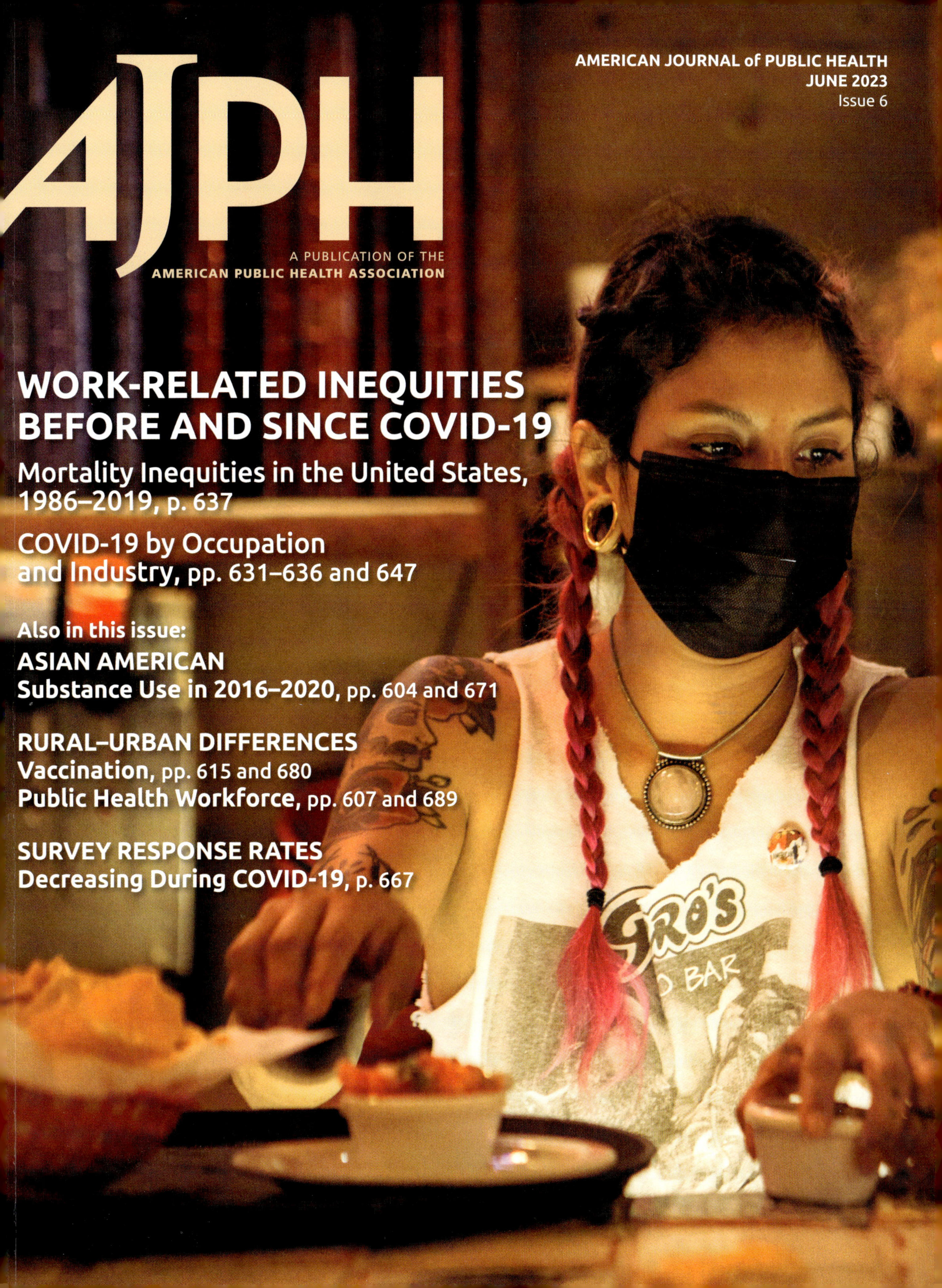

AMERICAN JOURNAL of PUBLIC HEALTH
JUNE 2023
Issue 6

AJPH

A PUBLICATION OF THE
AMERICAN PUBLIC HEALTH ASSOCIATION

WORK-RELATED INEQUITIES BEFORE AND SINCE COVID-19

Mortality Inequities in the United States, 1986–2019, p. 637

COVID-19 by Occupation and Industry, pp. 631–636 and 647

Also in this issue:

ASIAN AMERICAN
Substance Use in 2016–2020, pp. 604 and 671

RURAL–URBAN DIFFERENCES
Vaccination, pp. 615 and 680
Public Health Workforce, pp. 607 and 689

SURVEY RESPONSE RATES
Decreasing During COVID-19, p. 667

APHA
AMERICAN PUBLIC HEALTH ASSOCIATION
For science. For action. For health.

AJPH®, published monthly, is the official Journal of the American Public Health Association®, 800 I St NW, Washington, DC 20001-3710; (202) 777- APHA; TDD (202) 777-2500. APHA is a nongovernmental professional society founded in 1872, representing all disciplines and specialties in public health.

The *American Journal of Public Health*® (*AJPH*) (print ISSN: 0090-0036; electronic ISSN: 1541- 0048), first published in 1911, is the official journal of the American Public Health Association® (APHA). The oldest and largest organization of public health professionals in the world, APHA represents approximately 30 000 members from more than 50 occupations of public health.

Submissions: Visit www.editorialmanager.com/ajph or ajph.edmgr.com for online manuscript preparation and submission guidelines. Contributions of original unpublished research, social science analyses, scholarly essays, critical commentaries, departments, and letters to the editor are welcome. Questions? Write ajph.submissions@apha.org or call APHA at (202) 777-2469.

Print plus online subscriptions: Institutional price (print copy with online access for a single institution and all authorized users, regardless of geographic location) varies by size of organization and ranges from $993–$1445 for US organizations, and $1073–$1526 for international organizations (air delivery); multiple campuses not permitted without special arrangement. Details of the tiered pricing system at https://subscriptionoffice.com/pages/apha-landing-page. To order, write apha.subscriptions@apha.org.

Online only subscriptions: Institutional price for one institution and its authorized users (regardless of geographic location) is $878–$1307. To order, write apha.subscriptions@apha.org. For academic consortia or multisite corporate subscriptions, contact apha.subscriptions@apha.org.

Print-only subscriptions: Institutional price is US $701, $782 international.

Back print issues: A limited number of print issues are for sale. Single copies are US $49, $55 international (air delivery). Shipping included; prepay only. To order, write apha.subscriptions@apha.org.

Reprints: For prices and ordering information on 50 or more reprints, check the Reprints section at www.ajph.org. To order smaller quantities of reprints (rush delivery), use the "Purchase Article" link on the article site itself.

Electronic access: Online articles more than 10 years old are available free for personal use at www.ajph.org. Recent articles are available through pay-per-view: single PDF article for $24, single issue access for 24 hours for $33, or entire site access for 24 hours for $38.

Postal information: Periodicals postage paid at Washington, DC, and additional mailing offices. Postmaster: Send address changes to American Journal of Public Health, 800 I St NW, Washington, DC 20001-3710.

Address changes: Send to AJPH, Membership Department (members) or AJPH Subscriptions (subscribers), APHA, 800 I St NW, Washington, DC 20001-3710. Or write to membership.mail@apha. org (members) or apha.subscriptions@apha.org (subscribers).

Advertising: For pricing and other information, see www.ajph.org. Please write to ashell.alston@apha.org or call (202) 777-2470 for other advertising opportunities. Ask about special exhibit packages and sponsorships. Acceptance of advertising by the *Journal* does not imply endorsement of products.

Indexes: Publications that index or abstract articles from AJPH include the following: Ageline, Assia (Applied Social Science Index and Abstracts), Biological Abstracts, Chemical Abstracts, CINAHL, Criminal Justice Abstracts, EMBASE, EMCare, Environmental Abstracts, e-psyche, ERIC, ETOH (Alcohol and Alcohol Problems Science Database), Excerpta Medica, Food Science and Technology, General Science Index, Grateful Med, Hospital Literature Index, Human Resources Abstracts, International Pharmaceutical Abstracts (IPA), Medline, Physical Education Index, Pollution Abstracts, Psychological Abstracts, PsychINFO, Safety Science Abstracts, Sage Family Studies Abstracts, Sage Human Resources Abstracts, Science Citation Index, SCOPUS, SIIC Data Bases, Social Work Research and Abstracts, and Statistical Reference Index (SRI)/LexisNexis.

AJPH

A PUBLICATION OF THE
AMERICAN PUBLIC HEALTH ASSOCIATION

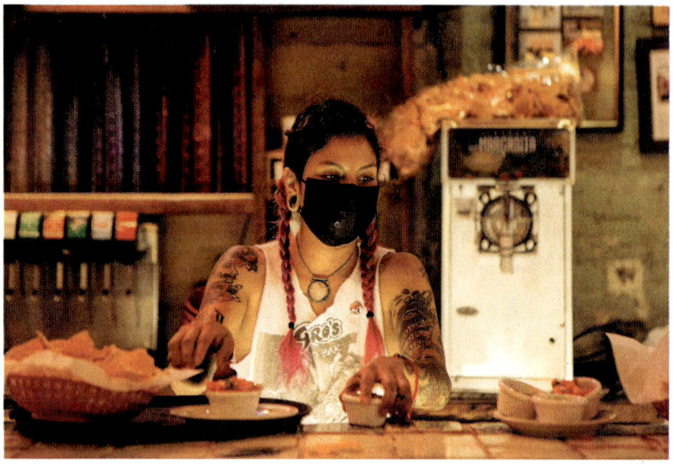

COVER: City of Austin Defies Governor on Mask Mandate. A server wearing a protective mask prepares an order at a taco bar in Austin, TX, on Wednesday, March 10, 2021. Texas Attorney General Ken Paxton blasted Austin officials and threatened to sue them for defying a statewide moratorium on rules forcing Texans to don face coverings in public, the *Washington Post* reported.

Cover concept and selection by Aleisha Kropf. Photograph by Mary Kang/Bloomberg via Getty Images. Printed with permission.

APHA
AMERICAN PUBLIC HEALTH ASSOCIATION
For science. For action. For health.

Promoting public health research, policy, practice, and education is the *AJPH* mission. As we widen our scope to embrace global issues, we also sharpen our focus to support the needs of public health practitioners. We invite contributions of original unpublished research, opinion and commentary, and letters to the editor.

The *Journal* is printed on acid-free recycled paper.

OPEN ACCESS ONLINE ONLY PODCAST DATA SUPPLEMENT AVAILABLE

EDITOR'S CHOICE

597 Bringing Workers Safety, Health, and Well-Being Front and Center in Public Health
A. Morabia

BOOKS & MEDIA

598 Documenting Our History, Protecting Our Futures: Queer Communities
M. Aaron Guest

601 A Food Politician Memoir and a Plea for Social Justice
S. Hercberg

OPINIONS, IDEAS, & PRACTICE

EDITORIALS

604 Health Equity Research: A Clarion Call to Focus on Racism, Not Race
E. Wu

607 Our Helpers Need Help: Challenges Faced by Rural Public Health Workers in the COVID-19 Pandemic
J. K. Harris

609 Looking Back: Does Social Capital Still Matter for Health? Revisiting Pearce and Davey Smith 20 Years On
M. McKee, M. Parbst, and D. Stuckler

612 The Short and the Long Arm of the COVID-19 Pandemic: Direct and Indirect Effects of the US Economic Lockdown
D. P. Do and R. Frank

615 Vaccine Uptake and Hesitancy in Rural America in the Wake of the COVID-19 Pandemic
T. Callaghan

618 Public Health Data of the People, by the People, for the People: A Public Health of Consequence, June 2023
F. Kapadia

PERSPECTIVES

620 Addressing the Need for Accountability in Public Health
S. A. Rasmussen, R. A. Goodman, and W. E. Parmet

NOTES FROM THE FIELD

623 Public Libraries for Public Health: COVID-19 Response Efforts in Prince George's County, Maryland
D. de Acosta, N. A. Brown, R. Zukowski, E. Mann, and E. Dawson-Hahn

627 The Chelsea Project: Turning Research and Wastewater Surveillance on COVID-19 Into Health Equity Action, Massachusetts, 2020–2021
C. Alonso, B. Keppard, S. Bates, D. Cortez, F. Amaya, and K. Dinakar

THE OCCUPATIONAL DIMENSION OF PUBLIC HEALTH

631 The Other Side of the Balance Sheet: Work as a Fundamental Determinant of Health
D. Hawkins

634 COVID-19 May Have Been Job Related for One Fourth of Diagnosed Adults
J. P. Leigh

RESEARCH & ANALYSIS

THE OCCUPATIONAL DIMENSION OF PUBLIC HEALTH

637 Dead Labor: Mortality Inequities by Class, Gender, and Race/Ethnicity in the United States, 1986–2019
J. Eisenberg-Guyot, M. C. Finsaas, and S. J. Prins

647 COVID-19 Risk by Workers' Occupation and Industry in the United States, 2020–2021
A. Gaffney, D. U. Himmelstein, D. McCormick, and S. Woolhandler

CLIMATE CHANGE

657 Excess Injury Mortality in Washington State During the 2021 Heat Wave
J. A. Casey, R. M. Parks, T. A. Bruckner, A. Gemmill, and R. Catalano

HISTORY

661 "Ashamed to Put My Name to It": Monsanto, Industrial Bio-Test Laboratories, and the Use of Fraudulent Science, 1969–1985
D. Rosner and G. Markowitz

SURVEILLANCE

667 Decreasing Survey Response Rates in the Time of COVID-19: Implications for Analyses of Population Health and Health Inequities
N. Krieger, M. LeBlanc, P. D. Waterman, S. L. Reisner, C. Testa, and J. T. Chen

OPEN-THEMED RESEARCH

671 Substance Use Among Asian American Adults in 2016–2020: A Difference-in-Difference Analysis of a National Survey on Drug Use and Health Data
Y. Yan, M. Yoshihama, J. S. Hong, and F. Jia

680 Rural–Urban Differences in Vaccination and Hesitancy Rates and Trust: US COVID-19 Trends and Impact Survey on a Social Media Platform, May 2021–April 2022
S. Soorapanth, R. Cheung, X. Zhang, A. H. Mokdad, and G. A. Mensah

689 Competencies, Training Needs, and Turnover Among Rural Compared With Urban Local Public Health Practitioners: 2021 Public Health Workforce Interests and Needs Survey
P. M. Kett, B. Bekemeier, D. G. Patterson, and K. Schaffer

BACKMATTER

OTHER DEPARTMENTS

704 Subscription Form

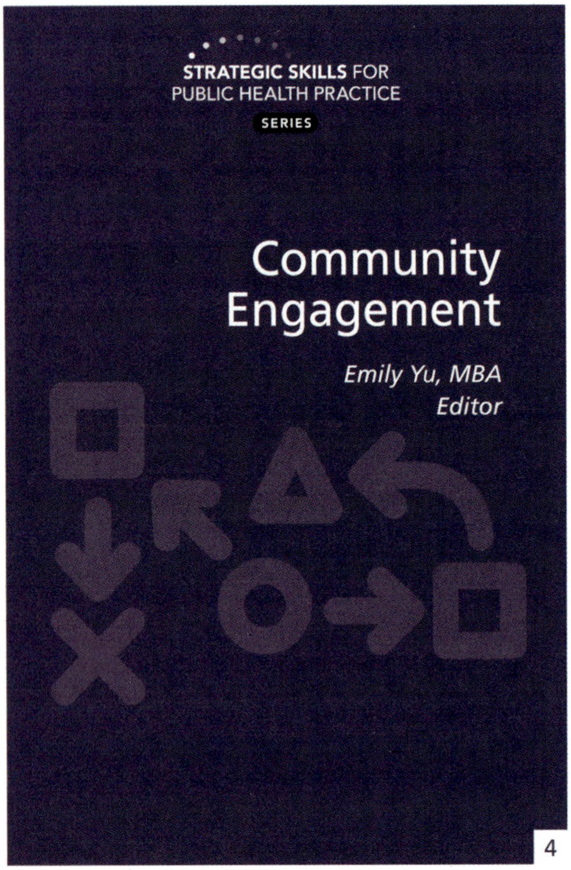

978-087553-3308, 108 PP, DIGITAL & SOFTCOVER

Community Engagement

Edited by Emily Yu, MBA

Community Engagement is the first book to be published from our new *Strategic Skills for Public Health Practice* series. This book brings the concept of community engagement to life through first-person stories, real-world examples and valuable insights from leaders across sectors. Curated specifically for public health practitioners and those interested in supporting community health, the book's chapters, guidance, and perspectives from the field will enhance readers' understanding of community-centered design and provide the tools to support organizational practices that drive better health for all.

APHABOOKSTORE.ORG

APHA PRESS

AN IMPRINT OF AMERICAN PUBLIC HEALTH ASSOCIATION

Bringing Workers Safety, Health, and Well-Being Front and Center in Public Health

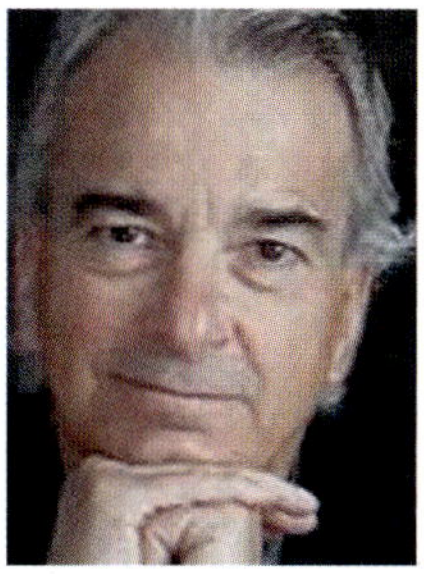

The importance of jobs, occupations, and work in people's health has been consistently stressed in this journal. This editorial reviews some of the milestone articles we have published since 2018 and presents two new articles from the current issue.

Emily Quinn Ahonen et al. described why work determined observed societal-level health inequities. She and her colleagues outlined the methodological challenges associated with incorporating work in the study of health inequities (https://bit.ly/3GgpTXm).

Paul A. Landsbergis et al. stressed the lack of adequate funding limiting the extent to which nuanced measures of work exposures are included in health surveillance systems. For example, the National Institute for Occupational Safety and Health budget pales in comparison with National Institutes of Health budgets, despite the fact that occupational injury has an economic burden similar to that of cancer or cardiovascular disease (https://bit.ly/3U9sHLt).

In 2020, David Michaels and Jordan Barab celebrated the 50th anniversary of the passage of the 1970 Occupational Safety and Health Act (OSHA), which contributed to a significant reduction in work-related deaths, injuries, and illnesses. Still, OSHA needs to be empowered and modernized to be able to prevent the millions of injuries and thousands of deaths among workers annually (https://bit.ly/3MfQ30j). As a case in point, the United States entered the COVID-19 pandemic without a workplace airborne disease standard, which would have helped to keep workers safe from the coronavirus. The project had started after the H1N1 influenza epidemic in 2009, but the administration in place in 2017 halted the adoption of the standards (https://bit.ly/3nIhkhy).

Meg Lovejoy et al. added that the COVID-19 health crisis revealed structural conditions that heightened the vulnerability of workers and their families to physical and psychosocial stressors. They proposed a model of work redesign updated for the 21st century, including increased worker schedule control and voice, moderated job demands, and enhanced social relations at work (https://bit.ly/3nEHq53). The redesign, Leslie Hammer wrote, should target the most vulnerable workers, and in particular women, who make up a majority of workers in low-wage jobs. The goal should be not only safety and health, but also bringing worker well-being and work redesign front and center in the 21st century (https://bit.ly/3m3siO8).

In this issue, we publish two analyses of the public health dimension of occupation based on data from the National Health Interview Survey (NHIS) before and since COVID-19. Jerzy Eisenberg-Guyot et al. use pre–COVID-19 data (up to 2019) to show that when occupations are categorized in terms of social classes, workers have a shorter longevity than their employers and other higher social class groups (p. 637). Adam Gaffney et al. use the 2020–2021 NHIS surveys to assess the differences in COVID-19 self-reported infections across occupational groups—finding, consistent with similar surveys in other countries, that workers having close contact with sick persons or the public are at greater risk (p. 647).

Editorialists Paul Leigh (p. 634) and Devan Hawkins (p. 631) describe the strengths and limitations of the NHIS data to assess the inequitable impact of COVID-19. Occupation health research faces methodological and financial difficulties that are reflected in these publications. Still, the inequities are so massive that they would most likely subsist if stricter assessment of confounding by age, gender, race/ethnicity, housing, crowding, and health status could have been factored in.

Most importantly, the fact that the NHIS and self-reported exposure are the best available measures to assess the impact of COVID-19 on occupational groups nationally is another expression of an essential deficiency of US public health: the lack of population-based health monitoring systems, as the ones described in the May issue of *AJPH* (https://bit.ly/3zz0WTj). Such systems, based on random sampling of the population, should be sufficiently granular to assess work-related differences and, during an epidemic, incorporate a seroprevalence component.

The articles mentioned here illustrate the numerous contributions in *AJPH* that stress the importance of jobs, occupations, and work in people's health. The pandemic has intensified their timeliness and the urgency of intervening on the public health dimension of work. AJPH

Alfredo Morabia, MD, PhD
Editor-in-Chief, AJPH

DOI: https://doi.org/10.2105/AJPH.2023.307304

59 Years Ago

Fifty Years of Occupational Health

When [Alice Hamilton] attended the Fourth International Congress on Occupational Accidents and Diseases at Brussels in 1910, she found that "for an American it was not an occasion for national pride." The Belgian representative disposed of American activity with the curt statement, "It is well known that there is no industrial hygiene in the United States. Ça n'existe pas." Since then major changes have taken place. Health problems arising out of exposure to noxious substances and dangerous working conditions have been recognized in numerous instances and measures have been taken to prevent or to ameliorate the effects resulting from such exposure. Reforms have been brought about by the joint efforts of organized labor, enlightened employers, physicians, legislators and community leaders. Prominent in this development from the beginning was the Division of Occupational Health of the U.S. Public Health Service. . . . [I]n 1914 . . . a dozen commissioned officers were assigned to study the health problems of miners, garment workers, steel workers, and other industrial groups. . . . Lead poisoning, silicosis, anthrax, industrial fatigue, dermatoses, illumination, the physiological effects of high temperatures—these and other problems were subjected to intensive investigation. Today, the Division of Occupational Health is continuing this tradition.

From AJPH, *November 1964, p. 1921*

107 Years Ago

Report of the Committee on Occupational Mortality

In a study of occupational mortality, the Committee believes it essential to include morbidity as related to occupation. A study of economic conditions and the slow working changes of physical and mental deterioration—the health hazards—due to occupational requirements and environment are essential to a profitable study of the problem, and these data can be obtained with completeness only during the lifetime of the patients. . . . [Q]uarrymen, certain groups of the textile workers, garment workers and others . . . show higher mortality rates for the working periods of life than do corresponding age groups of all occupied persons of the same sex. On further analysis, the higher mortality can be traced to a higher incidence from pulmonary tuberculosis. This is so constant over long periods of time and in different countries that we cannot escape the conclusion that the particular kind of work done by these groups carries with it a higher incidence of tuberculosis. What is thus indicated to be true of tuberculosis is probably true in varying degrees of a number of other diseases.

From AJPH, *January 1916, pp. 49–50*

Documenting Our History, Protecting Our Futures: Queer Communities

M. Aaron Guest, PhD, MPH, MSW

ABOUT THE AUTHOR

The author is with the Center for Innovation in Healthy and Resilient Aging, Edson College of Nursing and Health Innovation, Arizona State University, Phoenix.

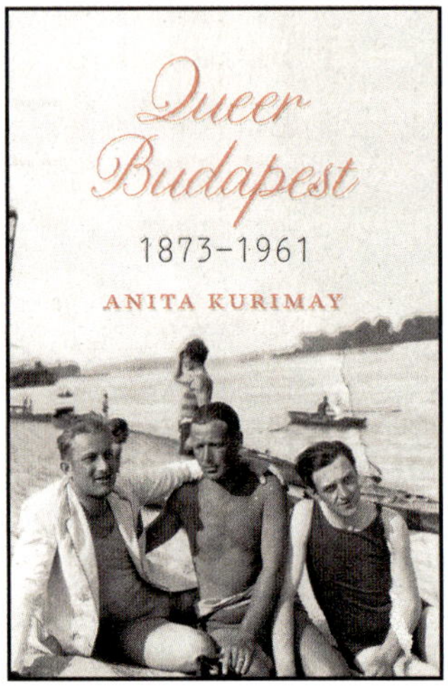

Queer Budapest, 1873–1961
By Anita Kurimay
336 pp.; $35.00 paper
Chicago, IL: University of Chicago Press; 2020
ISBN: 978-0226705798

The continued attacks on and demonization of lesbian, gay, bisexual, transgender, and queer (LGBTQ) people in the United States highlight the ongoing tension related to discussing, recognizing, and accepting sexual and gender identity in the United States. Often couched as a form of "protection" for the masses, these attacks present nonheterosexual sexuality and nonbinary gender as abnormal, something only recently discovered. Globally, these attacks gloss over the reality that nonheterosexual and nonbinary people have always existed. Yet, rarely have their stories been part of the historical record. What limited history exists is almost exclusively told from a Western European or North American framework. This is not meant to belittle the excellent scholarship of individuals such as Lilian Faderman (*The Gay Revolution: The Story of the Struggle*) and Peter Ackroyd (*Queer City: Gay London from the Romans to the Present Day*) but to recognize the gap in our collective history.[1,2]

Enter *Queer Budapest, 1873–1961* by Anita Kurimay. *Queer Budapest* weaves together a story that examines the complexity of nonnormative sexual or queer identity across time and sociopolitical changes. By exploring the end of the 19th century to the middle of the 20th century, Kurimay shows shifts in cultural and political thought on how queer men should be viewed, treated, and dealt with. The political, social, and judicial systems came into contact.

Supported by case examples of individuals who found themselves as part of these systems, she shows how the underhanded ambivalence, and perhaps even acceptance, of the late 19th century was replaced by the medicalization of queer identity after World War I, which gave way to outlawing as the communists rose to power.

Relying on archival research, historical documents, and contemporary sources, *Queer Budapest* is a refreshing take on the historical narrative format. Kurimay brings to life an overlooked time in Eastern Europe's and Hungary's history. In her telling, Budapest becomes not only a backdrop for these social and political changes but also an essential character. The city's role as the center of government and social life cannot be separated from the challenges faced by the individuals documented in the book. Men were attracted to the city as the social hub for queer identities, but they put themselves at a greater risk for arrest and the effects of changes in politics.

In this way, the book serves as an excellent companion piece to Beachey's *Gay Berlin: Birthplace of a Modern Identity*.[3] Both works situate the environment and culture of their respective cities as central to shaping the development of queer identities. Where *Queer Budapest* stands out is how Kurimay has situated Budapest as the urban center in contrast to the rural areas that surround it.

One of the significant tensions of the book is the role of the penal code, and eventually the homosexual registry, in criminalizing and ostracizing queer identities. The way a tool ostensibly for public health is so quickly corrupted and unevenly applied according to social class serves as a stark warning for the proposed anti-LGBTQ bills of today. However, the multitude of tensions highlight the complexity of challenges faced by sexual and gender minority and queer individuals. These include the tensions between the criminalization of queer men and the ambivalence toward queer women, the cultural understanding versus pathological assessment of same-sex behavior, the rural versus urban dichotomy, and the role of modernization in shaping queer identities.

TEXT STRUCTURE

Over an introduction and six chapters, Kurimay contemplates how behavior remains the same but society's treatment and understanding change. The introduction provides critical frameworks for reading the remaining chapters. Chapter 1 introduces the reader to Budapest and the treatment of queer identities in the late 19th century. Chapter 2, which examines the writings of journalists and others throughout Europe, takes us into the 20th century and points toward what could have been had peace prevailed. Chapter 3 highlights a forgotten time, the brief existence of the Hungarian Society Republic, which for a time adapted holistic means of understanding a person.

Chapter 4 takes an exciting turn, reviewing how society treated the divorce and libel trial of an influential woman accused of having a female lover. The reader is returned to 1920 in Chapter 5 and introduced to the coexistence of queer culture and identity and the politically conservative Hungarian regime. Finally, chapter 6 concludes with the entry of Hungary into World War II, the rise of the communist state, and the treatment of those with queer identities as enemies of the state.

HAVE WE LEARNED NOTHING? LESSONS FROM THE PAST

Kurimay has collected and documented the history of an overlooked population and provided us all a glimpse of the rich LGBTQ history still to tell. She has shifted the focus of LGBTQ history away from a solely Western European and North American view. She has introduced the rich role of Eastern Europe in the development of queer identities. She has developed an accessible, cohesive text that, for the most part, flows together. The subplot in chapter 4 briefly distracts from what seems to be the overarching aim of the book, although it does provide a meaningful context and comparison with the experiences of queer men. One is left wondering about the outcomes and lives of the many individuals described throughout the text. However, the lack of closure is a result of the historical record as opposed to a failing of the author.

There seems to be a missed opportunity to better link the past and present. Despite the official decriminalization in the 1960s, LGBTQ individuals in Hungary continue to face cultural and legal challenges. Hungary is regularly ranked at the bottom among European Union countries and most others in Eastern Europe with respect to LGBTQ rights and acceptance.[4] Although Hungary does have antidiscrimination laws, including laws related to sexual and gender identity, the constitution bans same-sex marriage.

Furthermore, changing of one's gender identity and joint adoption by same-sex partners are forbidden. Following an emerging trend among former Warsaw Pact countries, Hungary passed "antipromotion bills" that limit the depiction of LGBTQ individuals and information throughout the country.[5] How might the country's history have influenced the introduction of these bills? How can we understand their support given the country's history? Kurimay provides us the background, but it is up to us and others to bring it together.

Although *Queer Budapest* is not a traditional LGBTQ health or public health book, it is one I believe many would benefit from reading. It helps illuminate that to understand a phenomenon, we cannot look just at the service level. We must identify the political, cultural, and historical social determinants driving health. The book highlights how we must look to the past as we face today's battles. The criminalization of queer identities and the use of a police state to unevenly enforce laws are something we know all too well. The differences in acceptance and human rights of LGBTQ people according to the political party in power are experienced the world over. The role of a registry in managing and controlling the LGBTQ community is a stark reminder as we face the growing threat of registries to track individuals who are transitioning, drag queens, and even same-sex families. *Queer Budapest* is a biography of another place and time and an autobiography of our time. AJPH

CORRESPONDENCE

Correspondence should be sent to M. Aaron Guest, PhD, MPH, MSW, Center for Innovation in Healthy and Resilient Aging, Edson College of Nursing and Health Innovation, Arizona State University, 500 N 3rd St, Phoenix, AZ 85004 (e-mail: aaron.guest@asu.edu). Reprints can be ordered at http://www.ajph.org by clicking the "Reprints" link.

PUBLICATION INFORMATION

Full Citation: Guest MA. Documenting our history, protecting our futures: queer communities. *Am J Public Health*. 2023;113(6):598–600.

Acceptance Date: February 26, 2023.

DOI: https://doi.org/10.2105/AJPH.2023.307275

CONFLICTS OF INTEREST

The author reports no conflicts of interest.

REFERENCES

1. Faderman L. *The Gay Revolution: The Story of the Struggle*. New York, NY: Simon & Schuster; 2015.
2. Ackroyd P. *Queer City: Gay London from the Romans to the Present Day*. New York, NY: Abrams; 2018.
3. Beachy R. *Gay Berlin: Birthplace of a Modern Identity*. New York, NY: Knopf Doubleday Publishing Group; 2015.
4. European Commission. Discrimination in the European Union. Available at: https://europa.eu/eurobarometer/surveys/detail/2251. Accessed February 20, 2023.
5. Hopkins V. In Hungary, an embattled L.G.B.T.Q. community takes to the streets. Available at: https://www.nytimes.com/2021/07/24/world/europe/hungary-lgbtq-pride-march-orban.html. Accessed February 20, 2023.

A Food Politician Memoir and a Plea for Social Justice

Serge Hercberg, MD, PhD

ABOUT THE AUTHOR

The author is emeritus professor of nutrition, University Sorbonne Paris North, Bobigny, France.

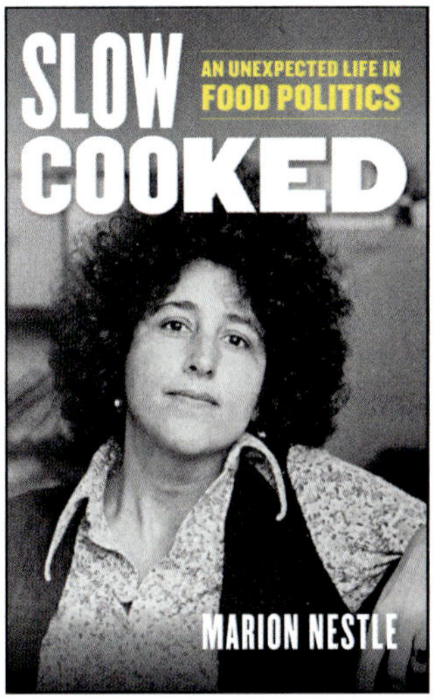

Slow Cooked: An Unexpected Life in Food Politics
By Marion Nestle
278 pp.; $29.95 hardcover
Berkeley, CA: University of California Press, 2022
ISBN: 0520384156

I thought I knew everything about the trials and tribulations of Marion Nestle, who today is considered to be the greatest warrior for public health nutrition in the United States. For more than 20 years, I have followed the many epic battles she has fought and continues to fight today: her battle against junk food, her denunciations of the influence of agri-food manufacturers on the nutrition and health of consumers and their ability to influence public policy, and her salutary questioning of the impact of conflicts of economic interest on recommendations and nutritional policies. Details can be found in her books, articles, and interviews and on her Web site. In short, I thought I knew everything about the career of Marion Nestle.

But her latest book, *Slow Cooked: An Unexpected Life in Food Politics*, reveals many other battles she led, of which the vast majority of her admirers were likely unaware. These very difficult, trying fights forged her personal and professional life and allow us to better understand what she has become today, in particular to better realize why her true career began after the age of 60 years: hence, the wonderful title of her book. Her story confirms that slow cooking often gives rise to the best, tastiest dishes.

This fascinating story of her life, told in the first person, reads like an adventure novel full of twists and turns. She teaches us about her long period of "simmering" with many obstacles to overcome, which made it possible to hatch this icon of nutrition who has inspired so many nutrition professionals worldwide. And I am one of those who have been deeply marked by her visions of nutrition and public health.

The first chapters remind us of the struggles of an American child born in the post-Depression period to a poor Jewish family who asks only to be recognized and loved, a sad and unfair childhood and a rather dark period but one fortunately interspersed with moments of joy, especially related to food. Her interests in food and the pleasures of eating in this dreary childhood undoubtedly weighed on her desire to study food a few years later.

We can follow her fight to escape her environment and to overcome the prejudices faced by women of her generation in the 1950s. As was expected at the time, she followed the societal model and left her studies to marry at 19 years of age and have two children she loved and cared for. However, a revelation came 10 years later. The story makes us relive the fight of a divorced woman with two children who decided to resume a university course.

It is in the bubbling context of this period marked by the struggles of civil rights movements that she earned a doctorate in molecular biology. But making a career in the world of science was not easy. We discover in detail the fight of a woman to have a professional career that recognized her skills and her work. It is also striking to find recurrently throughout her studies and later, in the different positions that she occupied in various structures, the same common threads: her constant interest

AJPH June 2023, Vol 113, No. 6

in (good) cuisine and (good) food and her passion for (good) nutrition.

It is also quite fascinating to see how she learned about this emerging discipline and became aware of its association with public health. In "on-the-job" training, she immersed herself in books and enriched herself through the various positive and negative encounters she had. Through her story, we discover the obstacles she had to overcome (and there were many) to evolve in an academic university setting still full of prejudice and social, religious, and racial discrimination.

By dint of persistence and despite the difficulties, she went on to a postdoctorate (in biochemistry) and became a lecturer and then an assistant professor. She was confronted with social inequalities (differences in wages between men and women, the difficulties of students from ethnic minority groups) but also discovered the pleasure and richness of teaching. First recruited as "her husband's wife" at the University of San Francisco, she had to overcome many obstacles to finally be named, on the basis of her skills, professor of biology and of nutritional sciences at the university.

Eventually, she decided to work as a senior nutrition policy advisor at the US Department of Health and Human Services. She spent two years there in what she describes as a federal prison, a very difficult experience for the rebel faced with the constraints of a Reagan era administration so close to economic actors and their political influences. She worked for a year and a half on the famous *Surgeon General's Report on Nutrition and Health*,[1] having to juggle between science and multiple pressures so as not to upset influential politicians who are so quick to relay the demands of economic actors. In the absence of being able to recommend reductions in meat consumption—a flagship of the American economy—it was necessary to limit herself to mentioning saturated fats, terminology better tolerated by meat producers. She saw from the inside the pressure from lobbies that relied on politicians to block any unwanted messages and any unwanted public health action that they considered to go against their interests.

After these two years within the "DC culture," she came out even better armed to testify against and denounce the interference of food industrialists. This provided her with the material to write books that became cult favorites and allowed her to be present in the media and listened to by health professionals as well as the general public. But it also gave her the desire to regain her total freedom by returning to the university setting. She was recruited by New York University, where she developed further, still having to overcome many obstacles, a nutrition department while pursuing (with great enthusiasm) a career as a critical analyst of food industry stocks.

She shares many "tasty" anecdotes that illustrate the underside of her new adventures and her meetings with scientists, cooks, public health officials, journalists, food columnists, politicians, and students, meetings that were often pleasant and sometimes rather unpleasant but that helped her to grow.

And we suddenly discover that it is not until the age of 66 years that she published her book *Food Politics*,[2] which marked a turning point in her life and made her the great lady who raised the concept of the link between food and politics. After the release of her book, she had to face attacks, criticisms, and even threats of lawsuits. She experienced moments of doubt but was encouraged by testimonials of recognition, multiple awards and prizes she received, and the attention of the media that opened their doors to her.

By telling us the story of her life, Marion Nestle allows us to understand the journey of a woman whose courage and perseverance led to the birth of a militant public health activist, but one who always knew how to rely on science and knowledge. She is a critical activist against those who, for the defense of purely economic interests, heavily influence the food and health of populations, those (in particular, food manufacturers) who want us to believe that nutritional problems are only a matter of individual responsibility, thus minimizing or even completely denying their influence on the food choices of consumers. She is an activist certainly, but a thousand miles from the image of an Ayatollesque hygienist that some want to give to nutritionists, reminding us that, on the contrary, pleasure and health are compatible and desirable in the field of food.

Moreover, this book, beyond the author's personal story and the issue of nutrition, is a magnificent plea for social justice against all types of discrimination and for the emancipation of women. She teaches us great lessons on how to overcome obstacles while maintaining intellectual integrity and faith in science and public health. Marion, thank you for your actions. Keep fighting and give us many more of the lessons of hope that inspire us so deeply. AJPH

CORRESPONDENCE

Correspondence should be sent to Serge Hercberg, MD, PhD, EREN, UFR SMBH, University Sorbonne Paris North, 74 rue Marcel Cachin, 93017 Bobigny, France (e-mail: hercberg@eren.smhh.univ-paris13.fr). Reprints can be ordered at http://www.ajph.org by clicking the "Reprints" link.

PUBLICATION INFORMATION

Full Citation: Hercberg S. A food politician memoir and a plea for social justice. *Am J Public Health*. 2023;113(6):601–603.

Acceptance Date: February 28, 2023.

DOI: https://doi.org/10.2105/AJPH.2023.307276

CONFLICTS OF INTEREST

The author reports no conflicts of interest.

REFERENCES

1. Dept of Health and Human Services (USDHHS): Public Health Service. *The Surgeon General's Report on Nutrition and Health*. Washington, DC: US Government Printing Office; 1988.
2. Nestle M. *Food Politics: How the Food Industry Influences Nutrition and Health*. Berkeley, CA: University of California Press, 2002.

Health Equity Research: A Clarion Call to Focus on Racism, Not Race

Elwin Wu, PhD

ABOUT THE AUTHOR

Elwin Wu is with the Social Intervention Group, Columbia School of Social Work, New York, NY.

See also Yan et al., p. 671.

There is a documented paucity of research regarding health inequities experienced by Asian Americans. The National Institutes of Health allocated 0.12% of its research budget on health inequities among Asian Americans from 1992 to 2000 and only 0.18% from 2000 to 2018.[1] This is in contrast to Asian Americans being the fastest growing major racial/ethnic group in the United States since 2000, nearly doubling in size in that time period and projected to exceed 46 million by 2060.[2]

In their article in this issue of *AJPH*, Yan et al. (p. 671) begin to fill this gap by reporting that the increase in substance use—specifically alcohol, cocaine, and tranquilizer use—during 2020 compared with 2016 to 2019 was significantly greater among Asian American relative to White American adults. This study used data from the National Survey on Drug Use and Health (NSDUH), arguably the leading source of data with respect to national trends on substance use in the United States. Yan et al. also increased the rigor of their findings via the use of propensity score weighting in the analytic approach, thus providing a more causally valid estimate of the difference in substance use trends that can be attributed to race.

At the same time, the causal inference approach reveals a problem of a fundamental nature. It should be obvious that race—that is, one's phenotype or even underlying genotype—cannot be and is not the actual cause of patterns of substance use, just like race itself cannot drive other prominent health inequities such as the disparate burden of HIV shouldered by Black populations in the United States.[3] If the causal factor for racial health disparities is not race, then what is? The answer is racism. This answer is so clear that racism has been put forth as a root cause of health inequities as well as a public health crisis.[4,5]

It is evident that Yan et al. are aware of this because they present anti-Asian racism as the impetus for the study and premise for the stated hypotheses. They articulate that the COVID-19 pandemic–driven increase in anti-Asian racism could drive increased substance use among Asian Americans during the 2020 time period during the COVID-19 pandemic versus the time period preceding COVID-19. Yet, the study by Yan et al. perpetuated the aforementioned fundamental problem that is too often present in racial health equity research: using race as a proxy for racism. In other words, their study did not directly test the putative cause (experiences of anti-Asian racism) of changes in substance use.

The NSDUH data set did not include measures of racism, prohibiting a direct test of the racism hypotheses. This problem is not unique to NSDUH. A recent environmental scan of public health surveillance and monitoring systems found that only three out of 125 of the systems collected data on individual experiences of racism and none directly collected data on other aspects of racism such as internalized or structural racism.[6]

CONSIDERATIONS FOR RACE AS A PROXY FOR RACISM

Yan et al. understandably saw race as the best proxy for racism in the NSDUH data set. However, by leaving that presumption unspoken, they effectively conflated race with racism. Furthermore, by not acknowledging this limitation in a study ostensibly about the impact of racism, Yan et al. implicitly perpetuate the acceptability of using race as a proxy for racism in health equity research. Even if one acknowledges and accepts using race as a proxy for racism, Yan et al. could still have reasonably tested the anti-Asian racism hypotheses with more rigor by also including comparisons to other non-White racial/ethnic populations (e.g., Black, Hispanic/Latine).

There are at least two ways that inclusion and comparison with these other populations provide additional tests of the anti-Asian racism mechanism posited by Yan et al. First, it allows one to see if the changes seen among Asians did or did not occur relative to other populations that experience racism but not anti-Asian racism (hence, no

COVID-19–related increase in racism exposure). Second, it allows for assessment into whether the drop in substance use among White Americans that appears to drive some of the significant difference-in-differences is a drop exhibited by all races/ethnicities other than Asian Americans or is specific to White Americans.

TOWARD ANTIRACIST RESEARCH

A focus on racism rather than race in the research enterprise is essential not only for documenting and understanding the impact of racism but also for efforts to intervene and remedy the impact of racism (i.e., antiracism). Antiracist research confronts and redresses the impact of racism both in the topics being studied as well as the research methods employed.[7] Consonant with antiracist research, moving from race to racism shifts the focus from people (e.g., White Americans [as perpetrators], people of color [as victims]) to dynamics and processes such as White supremacy and White supremacy culture that people are subjected to and shaped by. Decentering from Whiteness is a key component of antiracism. A recommendation for Yan et al. to include additional non-White racial/ethnic comparison groups is consonant with an antiracist approach to research because doing so moves away from using White Americans as the sole "reference" group.

THE FUTURE OF HEALTH EQUITY RESEARCH

Using race variables can indeed be useful for empirically establishing health inequities. Not only do Yan et al. bring attention to inequities faced by Asian Americans, but they also prompt attention to anti-Asian racism in the United States, which arguably has been downplayed historically compared with other groups in the United States to such an extent that anti-Asian racism can be seen as socially acceptable.[8,9] Concomitantly, a critical read of the study lays bare the value and necessity of utilizing measures of racism rather than relying on race as a proxy.

Public health research will benefit greatly when studies include assessment of the multiple forms and experiences of racism (e.g., interpersonal, internalized, institutional, structural, systemic). Using racism measures rather than racial categories can focus on the variance in racism experiences, which can provide key information on whether a change or difference in substance use on the order of 0.1 day per month seen in Yan et al. is clinically meaningful. The use of more nuanced measures of racism also neatly avoids one of the most pernicious limitations of using race as a proxy: aggregating and overlooking heterogeneity within a single designated racial group (e.g., grouping different Asians or Latine with an "Asian" or "Latine" designation, respectively).

Focusing on racism rather than race can usher in exciting new frontiers for research regarding the inequities faced by people of color. One example is intersectionality: utilizing measures of racism rather than race allows for analysis and elucidation of mechanisms (rather than just presence) of deleterious or buffering effects arising from intersectionality.[3,10] A second example is syndemics (the co-occurrence of multiple health and psychosocial problems that interact, generally reinforcing each other)[11]: racism as a public health problem suggests it could be added to the set of problems consisting of mental health, substance use, and HIV/AIDS[12] to further explain the disproportional prevalence and comorbidity experienced by sexual- and gender-expansive people of color. These are just two examples of the important and innovative scientific endeavors that can be undertaken if researchers heed the call of "racism, not race." AJPH

CORRESPONDENCE

Correspondence should be sent to Elwin Wu, Social Intervention Group, Columbia School of Social Work, 1255 Amsterdam Ave, New York, NY 10027 (e-mail: elwin.wu@columbia.edu). Reprints can be ordered at https://ajph.org by clicking the "Reprints" link.

PUBLICATION INFORMATION

Full Citation: Wu E. Health equity research: a clarion call to focus on racism, not race. *Am J Public Health.* 2023;113(6):604–606.

Acceptance Date: March 6, 2023.

DOI: https://doi.org/10.2105/AJPH.2023.307282

CONFLICTS OF INTEREST

The author has no conflicts of interest to declare.

REFERENCES

1. Đoàn LN, Takata Y, Sakuma K-LK, Irvin VL. Trends in clinical research including Asian American, Native Hawaiian, and Pacific Islander participants funded by the US National Institutes of Health, 1992 to 2018. *JAMA Netw Open.* 2019;2(7):e197432. https://doi.org/10.1001/jamanetworkopen.2019.7432
2. Budiman A, Ruiz NG. Key facts about Asian Americans, a diverse and growing population. Pew Research Center. Available at: https://www.pewresearch.org/fact-tank/2021/04/29/key-facts-about-asian-americans. Accessed February 28, 2023.
3. Wu E. Learning from "racism, not race" for intersectionality research and the research enterprise. *Soc Work Res* 2021;45(3):220–224. https://doi.org/10.1093/swr/svab014
4. Jones NL. Racism, a root cause of health inequity, must be tackled head on. *Am J Public Health.* 2020;110(9):1258–1259. https://doi.org/10.2105/AJPH.2020.305823
5. Andrews K. Racism is the public health crisis. *Lancet.* 2021;397(10282):1342–1343. https://doi.org/10.1016/S0140-6736(21)00775-3
6. White K, Beatty Moody DL, Lawrence JA. Integrating racism as a sentinel indicator in public health surveillance and monitoring systems. *Am J Public Health.* 2023;113(suppl 1):S80–S84. https://doi.org/10.2105/AJPH.2022.307160
7. Fleming PJ, Stone LC, Creary MS, et al. Antiracism and community-based participatory research:

synergies, challenges, and opportunities. *Am J Public Health.* 2023;113(1):70–78. https://doi.org/10.2105/AJPH.2022.307114

8. Kao AC. Invisibility of anti-Asian racism. *AMA J Ethics.* 2021;23(7):E507–E511. https://doi.org/10.1001/amajethics.2021.507
9. Man S. Anti-Asian violence and US imperialism. *Race Class.* 2020;62(2):24–33. https://doi.org/10.1177/0306396820949779
10. Bowleg L. Evolving intersectionality within public health: from analysis to action. *Am J Public Health.* 2021;111(1):88–90. https://doi.org/10.2105/AJPH.2020.306031
11. Singer M, Bulled N, Ostrach B, Mendenhall E. Syndemics and the biosocial conception of health. *Lancet.* 2017;389(10072):941–950. https://doi.org/10.1016/S0140-6736(17)30003-X
12. Stall R, Friedman M, Catania JA. Interacting epidemics and gay men's health: a theory of syndemic production among urban gay men. In: Wolitski RJ, Stall R, Valdiserri RO, eds. *Unequal Opportunity: Health Disparities Affecting Gay and Bisexual Men in the United States.* New York, NY: Oxford University Press; 2008: 251–274.

Our Helpers Need Help: Challenges Faced by Rural Public Health Workers in the COVID-19 Pandemic

Jenine K. Harris, PhD

ABOUT THE AUTHOR

Jenine K. Harris is in the public health program with the Brown School, Washington University in St. Louis, MO.

See also Kett et al., p. 689.

Implementation of effective public health programs and financial investment in local public health improves health and reduces mortality.[1,2] Despite this, and while the US population continues to grow, the full-time workforce at local health departments (LHDs) in the United States declined from 162 000 to 136 000 in the decade preceding the COVID-19 pandemic (2008–2019). As of 2019, there were no signs of the LHD workforce decline slowing, with 24% of the workforce planning to leave within the next year and 22% of health department staff planning to retire from their organization by 2023.[3] With flat funding and a declining workforce, in 2018, 20% of LHDs reported reducing at least one of six clinical and preventive services (i.e., immunization, maternal and child health, and screenings for high blood pressure, diabetes, blood lead, and communicable diseases; https://bit.ly/3TMdqQI).

RESPONDING TO COVID-19 WITH LIMITED RESOURCES

It was on this strained foundation that public health professionals at LHDs and other organizations across the country built COVID-19 surveillance and contact tracing programs; established and coordinated testing sites and programs; worked to ensure there were enough tests and personal protective equipment; implemented vaccine programs; developed pandemic policies and guidelines like social distancing, quarantine, and reopening businesses; collaborated with new and existing stakeholders; and communicated with the public about all of these things.

To complete this important and emergent work, LHDs repurposed internal resources that had been designated for other public health activities toward pandemic response. Perhaps the biggest shift of LHD resources was in staffing; 76% of LHD staff worked on pandemic response, leaving 24% of LHD staff working on nonpandemic activities and services.[4] State and local health departments hired new staff, with 17% of staff being hired during the pandemic.[4] Although the new staff eventually reduced the workload, the process of hiring and training a large number of new workers was yet another added task for health departments, especially early in the pandemic.

In addition to the increased COVID-19–related workload, public health professionals were regularly undermined by politicians[5] and challenged by widespread misinformation campaigns[6] disputing pandemic-related public health messaging and measures. Rural areas are more politically conservative than urban areas, and much of the politicized COVID-19 information and misinformation targeted conservatives, resulting in more spread and adoption of COVID-19 misinformation in rural areas.[7,8] Conservative political leaders were less likely to implement mitigation policies (e.g., social distancing), and conservatives were less likely to follow COVID-19 public health measures and mandates.[8] People living in US counties with a higher percentage of Republican votes in 2020 were vaccinated for COVID-19 at lower rates and died at higher rates in the year after vaccines became available.[8] Already facing a double disparity of poor health behaviors and outcomes in their communities and limited investment in rural public health before COVID-19,[9] the workforce in rural health departments had to face COVID-19 in communities with high levels of distrust of pandemic information and limited support from political leaders and constituents for mitigation efforts.[8,10]

COMPARING THE RURAL AND URBAN PUBLIC HEALTH WORKFORCES

Nearly half (44%) of LHDs in the United States serve rural jurisdictions that are home to about 65 million people or 20% of the US population. Although rural LHDs exist in a very different public health and political context than urban LHDs, workforce research has focused more on urban and suburban LHDs. Kett et al. (p. 689), published in this issue of *AJPH*, set out to fill this gap by comparing the rural and urban health department workforce during the COVID-19 pandemic to identify strengths and needs and to assess well-being. Kett et al. confirmed that professionals in rural LHDs have higher proficiency in community engagement and in building cross-sector partnerships compared with urban health departments. This has been reported in previous studies and is a necessity that permits rural health departments to leverage local connections and provide essential services, even with fewer staff and smaller budgets.[9]

However, Kett et al. may be the first to quantify the specific consequences for the well-being of rural public health professionals who had to continue to cultivate and rely on local partnerships in the extremely politically charged climate of public health during COVID-19. Specifically, for public health professionals who were not retiring but did intend to leave in the next year, Kett et al. reported statistically significantly higher odds of rural public health professionals being bullied or harassed because of their job compared with urban public health professionals. Compared with their urban counterparts, Kett et al. also reported that rural public health workers had statistically significantly higher odds of stress and of avoiding situations that made them think about COVID-19 (a possible symptom of posttraumatic stress disorder). While not included in results of the study by Kett et al., the 2021 Public Health Workforce Interests and Needs Survey data suggest that rural health departments had a higher percentage (35%) of staff agreeing that "I have felt my public health expertise was undermined or challenged by individuals outside of the health department" compared with the percentage of staff agreeing with this statement in urban health departments (28%).[10]

STRENGTHENING THE RURAL PUBLIC HEALTH WORKFORCE

COVID-19 is unlikely to be the last pandemic, and political polarization in the United States is not abating, although perhaps it will in the future. For the sake of the health of people living in rural areas and the well-being of rural public health workers, evidence from Kett et al. suggests a need for public health to focus on the hard work of changing its reputation in rural communities. A recent commentary on strategies to strengthen rural public health suggests four ways to start: (1) cultivate community-engaged partnerships before the next public health emergency, (2) include people from rural communities in the scientific and health care workforce, (3) include rural perspectives in public health intervention research, and (4) work on new health care service delivery models to meet rural needs.[11] The rural public health workforce is an important resource for protecting and improving public health across the United States and warrants investment. AJPH

CORRESPONDENCE

Correspondence should be sent to Jenine K. Harris, One Brookings Drive, Brown School, Washington University in St. Louis, St. Louis, MO 63130 (e-mail: harrisj@wustl.edu). Reprints can be ordered at https://ajph.org by clicking the "Reprints" link.

PUBLICATION INFORMATION

Full Citation: Harris JK. Our helpers need help: challenges faced by rural public health workers in the COVID-19 pandemic. *Am J Public Health*. 2023; 113(6):607–608.

Acceptance Date: March 19, 2023.

DOI: https://doi.org/10.2105/AJPH.2023.307297

ACKNOWLEDGMENTS

Thanks to Katie Stamatakis and Kristen Ruckdashel for reading a draft and making suggestions that improved the editorial and to Jonathon P. Leider for being a cool dude.

CONFLICTS OF INTEREST

The author has no conflicts of interest.

REFERENCES

1. Leider JP, Alfonso N, Resnick B, Brady E, McCullough JM, Bishai D. Assessing the value of 40 years of local public expenditures on health. *Health Aff (Millwood)*. 2018;37(4):560–569. https://doi.org/10.1377/hlthaff.2017.1171
2. Brown TT, Martinez-Gutierrez MS, Navab B. The impact of changes in county public health expenditures on general health in the population. *Health Econ Policy Law*. 2014;9(3):251–269. https://doi.org/10.1017/S1744133114000024
3. Sellers K, Leider JP, Gould E, et al. The state of the US governmental public health workforce, 2014–2017. *Am J Public Health*. 2019;109(5):674–680. https://doi.org/10.2105/AJPH.2019.305011
4. McCullough JM, Robins M. The opportunity cost of COVID for public health practice: COVID-19 pandemic response work and lost foundational areas of public health work. *J Public Health Manag Pract*. 2023;29(suppl 1):S64–S72. https://doi.org/10.1097/PHH.0000000000001656
5. Altheide DL. Pandemic in the time of Trump: digital media logic and deadly politics. *Symbolic Interact*. 2020;43(3):514–540. https://doi.org/10.1002/symb.501
6. van der Linden S. Misinformation: susceptibility, spread, and interventions to immunize the public. *Nat Med*. 2022;28(3):460–467. https://doi.org/10.1038/s41591-022-01713-6
7. Traberg CS, van der Linden S. Birds of a feather are persuaded together: perceived source credibility mediates the effect of political bias on misinformation susceptibility. *Pers Individ Dif*. 2022;185:111269. https://doi.org/10.1016/j.paid.2021.111269
8. Sehgal NJ, Yue D, Pope E, Wang RH, Roby DH. The association between COVID-19 mortality and the county-level partisan divide in the United States: study examines the association between COVID-19 mortality and county-level political party affiliation. *Health Aff (Millwood)*. 2022;41(6):853–863. https://doi.org/10.1377/hlthaff.2022.00085
9. Harris JK, Beatty K, Leider JP, Knudson A, Anderson BL, Meit M. The double disparity facing rural local health departments. *Annu Rev Public Health*. 2016;37(1):167–184. https://doi.org/10.1146/annurev-publhealth-031914-122755
10. de Beaumont Foundation and Association of State and Territorial Health Officials. Public Health Workforce Interest and Needs Survey: 2021 dashboard. 2022. Available at: https://phwins.org/national. Accessed March 9, 2023.
11. Lister JJ, Joudrey PJ. Rural mistrust of public health interventions in the United States: a call for taking the long view to improve adoption. *J Rural Health*. 2023;39(1):18–20. https://doi.org/10.1111/jrh.12684

Looking Back: Does Social Capital Still Matter for Health? Revisiting Pearce and Davey Smith 20 Years On

Martin McKee, DSc, Matthew Parbst, MA, and David Stuckler, PhD

ABOUT THE AUTHORS

Martin McKee is with the London School of Hygiene & Tropical Medicine, London, UK. Matthew Parbst is with the University of Toronto, Toronto, Canada. David Stuckler is with the University of Bocconi, Milan, Italy.

Twenty years ago, Pearce and Davey Smith asked, in an article in this journal, "Is social capital the key to inequalities in health?"[1] This was the latest salvo in what was becoming a heated argument between advocates of different explanations of the health of populations.

ARGUMENT AND COUNTERARGUMENT

Many thousands of words have been written on either side, and the literature is replete with nuance; therefore, in a short article such as this, it is necessary to (over)simplify the arguments.

On the one side are those who emphasized the position that individuals occupy in the social hierarchy and the psychological effects that flow from it; an example is Wilkinson, who saw inequality as having an impact on health that goes beyond that of conventional risk factors.[2] These researchers pointed to evidence that communities enjoyed better health if they had high levels of civic participation, reciprocity, and trust—things that facilitate cooperation for mutual benefit. It followed from this research that policymakers might improve health by measures that strengthened these attributes within communities—in other words, increased their social capital. An extreme version of this position was advanced by Putnam, a political scientist whose early work highlighted the importance of trust and reciprocity in explaining differences in the effectiveness of public administration in Italian regions. Although he at first dismissed the application of his ideas to health determinants, he changed his mind as the volume of literature showing an association accumulated, writing that if "you smoke and belong to no [social] groups, it's a toss-up statistically whether you should stop smoking or start joining [such groups]."[3(p331)]

Pearce and Davey Smith took an opposing view. In their 2003 article, they questioned what they described as a "vague, popular concept," launching a series of critiques. First, they asked how strong the evidence linking social capital and health actually was, noting it was often conflicting. They were particularly critical of studies across relatively large populations, such as American states or entire countries (e.g., Wilkinson[4]). They noted that many determinants of, for example, mortality in populations on this scale act over various durations and along different causal pathways, making it difficult to isolate the effect of one determinant and, especially, to ascertain causality. Second, they questioned whether there is clarity about what social capital is and how it should be measured, arguing that it has been defined "to include virtually all socioeconomic aspects of society."[1(p125)] Third, they raised doubts about the hypothesized pathways suggested as linking social capital and health. There are several, but those that exercised Pearce and Davey Smith most were psychological factors, and in particular the idea that a perceived low position in the social hierarchy is associated with negative emotions that feed into poor health. Fourth, they questioned whether the inability of conventional risk factors, measured in adulthood, to explain health inequalities was really so mysterious, noting the importance of insights from life course epidemiology, whereby exposures *in utero* or childhood cause disease decades later. Finally, they questioned whether social capital has any place in a discussion of the determinants of health, arguing that "much of what [Putnam] says with respect to health makes no epidemiological sense."[1(p127)]

Their main concern, however, related to the implications of research invoking social capital as a determinant of health. Logically, if the problems are low levels of trust and civic engagement, then policies to improve health should include measures designed to increase them. Although Pearce and Davey Smith accepted that such measures have benefits

AJPH June 2023, Vol 113, No. 6

in their own right, for the reasons listed here and others included in their article, they contended that the idea that they will improve health is simply a hypothesis. More importantly, they contended that focusing on these could divert attention from more important policies, especially those that improve human capital (e.g., through education) or economic capital (through redistribution of wealth). Worse, they argued, a focus on what disadvantaged communities can do for themselves, rather than addressing the structural reasons for their plight, is a form of victim-blaming at the community level.

So why do these distinguished scholars take such differing views? At least part of the problem is that it is often unclear what those working in this field are studying. In 1916, Hanifan proposed that interactions based on goodwill, fellowship, and mutual sympathy led to the accumulation of "social capital," which satisfied the social needs of both the individuals involved and the whole community.[5] There are, however, differing views of which of these levels is more important. Is it primarily an attribute of the individual or of the community, or of both? The main advocate of the former interpretation is Bourdieu, who saw the benefits that can accrue to someone as a consequence of their social networks but argued that these benefits are realized by virtue of the power that they can exert within those networks.[6] This power is, however, determined by context and, in particular, structures that confer advantage and related social norms. Others, comprising most writing on social capital, saw it as primarily acting at higher levels than the individual. Putnam, who as we saw was criticized by Pearce and Davey Smith, saw social capital as "features of social organizations, such as networks, norms and trust that facilitate action and cooperation for mutual benefit."[7(p35)]

The consequence of this terminological variation is that the instruments used to measure social capital vary greatly. They include those measured at the individual level, such as trust, interactions with others, or social support, and those at the community level, such as voter turnout or civic participation.

Despite the often heated rhetoric, some have questioned whether the two sides really were so far apart. Szreter and Woolcock, writing a year after Pearce and Davey Smith, sought to reconcile these positions.[8] They argued that it was impossible to ignore what was even then a large volume of research finding positive associations between diverse aspects of health and different measures of social capital. In subsequent years this body of literature has expanded. In 2020, Shiell et al. identified 28 systematic reviews published since Pearce and Davey Smith's review.[9] Although they examined different settings, age groups, and health outcomes, all but one found positive associations with at least one aspect of health, even if the results were sometimes inconsistent.

CURRENT STATE AND FUTURE DIRECTIONS

So where are we now with social capital and health? This was the subject of a theme issue of *Social Science and Medicine* published in 2020,[10] although the essential elements of its conclusions were already set out by Szreter and Woolcock 16 years earlier.[8] Pearce and Davey Smith were right to say that social capital is not *the* key to health inequalities. But it does play a role. Arguably, the differing views can be understood by reference to Isaiah Berlin's invocation of the ancient Greek poem in which "a fox knows many things, but a hedgehog knows one big thing." Some people look for a single overriding explanation of a phenomenon whereas others seek many different ones. Yet, although there are examples that come close to the former view, the suggestion that social capital's strongest advocates see it as the main determinant of health inequalities, as implied by the title of Pearce and Davey Smith's article, is something of a caricature. Most people accept that a mix of factors contribute, even if they disagree about how much. As Shiell et al. noted, what we do know about the link between social capital and health is, "it depends."[9(p4)]

We can draw five broad conclusions. First, the effects of social capital depend on context. Cognitive and structural elements of social capital, such as perceptions of trust, reciprocity, norms, and values and the quantity of relationships and memberships in institutions that can bring people together, often predict good health. So too do bonding and bridging forms.[11] This complexity calls for analytic designs that take account of the nature of these relationships, including the multilevel models used by Subramanian et al.[12]

Second, the effects of social capital may differ for group insiders, outsiders, and society as a whole. More complex research designs are needed to quantify exposures of neighbors and surrounding communities to better identify how an individual is situated within the group and relative to the dominant norms.

Third, the power of social capital may be less a matter of social capital per se than of its relationship with other health determinants. Recent scholarship has suggested that higher social capital has helped mitigate the risks to mental health associated with job loss.[13]

Fourth, we need more intervention studies on social capital and health.[14] Finally, research on social capital needs multidisciplinary research, but the irony is that this requires mutual trust and respect, often seemingly unattainable by those who study this phenomenon. AJPH

CORRESPONDENCE

Correspondence should be sent to Martin McKee, 15-17 Tavistock Place, London WC1H 9SH, United Kingdom (e-mail: martin.mckee@lshtm.ac.uk). Reprints can be ordered at http://www.ajph.org by clicking the "Reprints" link.

PUBLICATION INFORMATION

Full Citation: McKee M, Parbst M, Stuckler D. Looking back: does social capital still matter for health? revisiting Pearce and Davey Smith 20 years on. *Am J Public Health*. 2023;113(6): 609–611.

Acceptance Date: March 15, 2023.

DOI: https://doi.org/10.2105/AJPH.2023.307292

CONTRIBUTORS

M. McKee prepared the first draft, which all authors revised.

ACKNOWLEDGMENTS

D. Stuckler is funded by a European Research Council grant.

CONFLICTS OF INTEREST

The authors have no conflicts of interest to declare.

REFERENCES

1. Pearce N, Davey Smith G. Is social capital the key to inequalities in health? *Am J Public Health*. 2003; 93(1):122–129. https://doi.org/10.2105/AJPH.93.1.122
2. Wilkinson RG. *Unhealthy Societies: The Afflictions of Inequality*. London, UK: Routledge; 2002.
3. Putnam RD. *Bowling Alone: The Collapse and Revival of American Community*. New York, NY: Simon & Schuster Paperbacks; 2000.
4. Wilkinson R. Commentary: liberty, fraternity, equality. *Int J Epidemiol*. 2002;31(3):538–543. https://doi.org/10.1093/ije/31.3.538
5. Hanifan LJ. The rural school community center. *Ann Am Acad Pol Soc Sci*. 1916;67(1):130–138. https://doi.org/10.1177/000271621606700118
6. Wacquant LJ, Bourdieu P. *An Invitation to Reflexive Sociology*. Cambridge, UK: Polity; 1992.
7. Putnam R. The prosperous community: social capital and public life. *The American Prospect*. 1993;4:35–42.
8. Szreter S, Woolcock M. Health by association? Social capital, social theory, and the political economy of public health. *Int J Epidemiol*. 2004; 33(4):650–667. https://doi.org/10.1093/ije/dyh013
9. Shiell A, Hawe P, Kavanagh S. Evidence suggests a need to rethink social capital and social capital interventions. *Soc Sci Med*. 2020;257:111930. https://doi.org/10.1016/j.socscimed.2018.09.006
10. Moore S, Carpiano RM. Introduction to the special issue on "social capital and health: what have we learned in the last 20 Years and where do we go from here?" *Soc Sci Med*. 2020;257:113014.
11. Ehsan A, Klaas HS, Bastianen A, Spini D. Social capital and health: a systematic review of systematic reviews. *SSM Popul Health*. 2019;8:100425.
12. Subramanian SV, Kim DJ, Kawachi I. Social trust and self-rated health in US communities: a multilevel analysis. *J Urban Health*. 2002;79(4 suppl 1): S21–S34.
13. Reeves A, McKee M, Gunnell D, et al. Economic shocks, resilience, and male suicides in the Great Recession: cross-national analysis of 20 EU countries. *Eur J Public Health*. 2015;25(3):404–409.
14. Villalonga-Olives E, Wind TR, Kawachi I. Social capital interventions in public health: a systematic review. *Soc Sci Med*. 2018;212:203–218.

The Short and the Long Arm of the COVID-19 Pandemic: Direct and Indirect Effects of the US Economic Lockdown

D. Phuong Do, PhD, and Reanne Frank, PhD

ABOUT THE AUTHORS

D. Phuong Do is with the Zilber School of Public Health, University of Wisconsin-Milwaukee. Reanne Frank is with the Department of Sociology and the Institute for Population Research, Ohio State University, Columbus.

AJPH June 2023, Vol 113, No. 6

During the early months of the COVID-19 pandemic in the United States, as states began to implement business shutdowns to slow the spread of severe acute respiratory syndrome coronavirus 2 (SARS-CoV-2), Baker provided a dire estimate that 75% of US workers were employed in non-telework-friendly occupations and likely to either lose their job or risk exposure to SARS-CoV-2 at their workplace.[1] As highlighted by Baker, the group least likely to be able to work from home—characterized as workers whose interactions with the public are essential—was estimated to earn the lowest mean annual income, approxi mately $34 000 versus $66 000 for the most telework-friendly occupational group. This included workers in the retail, food service, beauty services, protective services, and transportation sectors.

INEQUITABLE BURDENS

Baker's projection—that unemployment risk from the COVID-19-induced shutdown was highest among the most economically vulnerable—was indeed realized. Jobs in the lowest-paying industries represented 30% of all jobs but accounted for almost 60% of jobs lost between February 2020 and October 2021.[2] Those forced to select financial viability over sheltering in place faced elevated risks as they reported to work, with calamitous consequences. Toward the end of the first year of the pandemic (December 2020), frontline workers were 20% more likely to test positive for SARS-CoV-2 than nonfrontline workers.[3] Those in the food processing industry had the highest elevated risk, with 45% higher odds of ever having tested positive.[3] This pattern of exposure extended to mortality; workers in the accommodation and food services industry had nearly twice the COVID-19 death rate of workers overall and almost three times the rate of those in nonessential industries.[4]

Although inability to telework was clearly correlated with economic vulnerability, the striking stratification of the US labor force could just as easily be demarcated by other familiar taxonomies underlying the country's social structure, notably race/ethnicity. The overrepresentation of racial/ethnic minorities in low-paying essential or frontline occupations foreshadowed the glaring inequitable burden and risks the lockdown would engender.

DISPROPORTIONATE HEALTH EFFECTS BY RACE/ETHNICITY

As of October 2022, age-adjusted mortality rates among Hispanics and non-Hispanic Blacks were 7.9 and 8.8 percentage points, respectively, above their percentage representation in the US population. By contrast, non-Hispanic Whites had a mortality advantage of 14.6 percentage points.[5] Copious commentaries have postulated that the disproportionate representation in telework-unfriendly occupations, particularly lower-standing positions associated with a high risk of exposure, was a key driver of the excess COVID-19 case and mortality burdens among racial/ethnic minorities.

Although studies directly examining the role of occupation in generating racial/ethnic disparities in COVID-19 cases and deaths remain limited, multiple indirect connections have been documented: (1) workplace outbreaks erupted in industries in which racial/ethnic minorities are overrepresented, (2) per capita COVID-19 mortality disparities between essential and nonessential workers are estimated to be largest among non-Hispanic Black and Hispanic workers, and (3) racial/ethnic minorities are disproportionately represented in occupations with higher COVID-19 case and death rates.[6] These observations, coupled with similar case fatality rates across race/ethnicity, are consistent with the hypothesis that occupation was a key (although by no means only) factor generating excess COVD-19 burdens in racial/ethnic minority communities.

THE LONG ARM OF COVID-19

As predicted by Baker, lower-income workers bore the brunt of the sudden and large economic shock brought on by the pandemic lockdown. In contrast to high-wage workers, whose employment rates remained virtually unchanged from February 2020 to February 2021, lower-income workers experienced an 11.7% decline in employment.[7] Those who were unable to work because of the pandemic struggled to meet their basic needs, as evidenced by their substantially higher prevalence of food insecurity: 16.4% in December 2020, as compared with only 4.2% among those who were able to keep their jobs.[8]

Compounding the economic hardship, many Americans were faced with increased responsibility for caregiving, not only for sick family or household members but also for children as the result of school and day-care closures across the country. This added burden hit workers without sick leave and women (who disproportionately shoulder the responsibility of caregiving) the hardest. Emerging evidence indicates that the additional caregiving burden led to lowered productivity among women in comparison with men, resulting in possible setbacks in terms of career progression and future earnings.[9] In the midst of these stressors generated from the shutdown, the United States saw a 9% increase in domestic violence.[10]

Economic losses among business owners were also unprecedented, with 22% closing doors in the first months of the pandemic.[11] Partly because of differences in demographic distributions across industries, racial/ethnic minority business owners disproportionately suffered; during the initial shutdown from February to April 2020, 41%, 32%, and 26% of the small businesses that stopped operating were Black, Hispanic, and Asian owned, respectively, as compared with 17% of those owned by White Americans, who make up 70% of business owners.[11]

The COVID-19-induced shutdown also affected children. The proportion of US households with children that were food insecure increased for the first time since 2011.[8] Furthermore, school closures represented an unprecedented disruption to children's education and development, particularly for students from families of lower socioeconomic status. Those in high-poverty districts lost an equivalent of 66% of a year's worth of achievement growth in math, as compared with 45% among students in low-poverty districts.[12]

POLICY RESPONSES

Few anticipated the depth and duration of the COVID-19 shutdown and its sweeping effects on income, education, familial responsibilities, and the very social fabric of society. Policy responses were exceptional in magnitude and depth. The Coronavirus Aid, Relief, and Economic Security (CARES) Act provided 80% of displaced workers more in benefits than they would have otherwise earned from work, resulting in a decrease in income inequality in 2020 relative to 2019.[13] The expanded child tax credit reduced child poverty and childhood food insecurity by approximately 30% and 26%, respectively, alleviating the elevated rates observed earlier in the pandemic.[14,15] In addition, the Families First Coronavirus Response Act required employers with fewer than 500 workers (representing more than 99% of US businesses) to provide workers with paid sick leave or expanded family leave for COVID-19-related reasons.

Furthermore, health care services related to COVID-19, including tests and vaccines, were covered by the federal government, effectively providing free access to COVID-19 care. Baker argued that the outcomes of vulnerable workers would depend, in part, on whether workplace protections and related policies were enacted. These safety net expansions, among others, helped to mitigate the worst possible outcomes of the pandemic.

That our country's most vulnerable experienced the brunt of the pandemic's detrimental effects was not a surprise. However, few had predicted the extent to which advantaged groups would benefit. Investors in the country's largest companies saw their wealth rise by more than a trillion dollars during the pandemic, and higher income workers now enjoy increased flexibility in the workplace with teleworking options.[13]

In contrast, lower-income workers have returned to prepandemic levels of economic precarity, living paycheck to paycheck with inadequate access to health care and no paid sick leave as expanded protections recede. Most of the federal protection programs have now ended, leaving many lower-income workers and their families at continued risk. Health care costs associated with COVID-19, including vaccinations, will likely no longer be covered by the US government once the current federally purchased supply is spent. The Families First Coronavirus Response Act expired at the end of 2020, and the expanded child tax credit and earned income tax credits have also lapsed. Paid sick leave is now neither required nor covered by the federal government.

LOOKING AHEAD

Barring new variants of concern, the current public health threat from COVID-19 has been greatly reduced in the face of widespread vaccination and decreased fatality rates. The US economy and daily life are slowly returning to their prepandemic states. However, the structural factors that engendered the gross inequities exposed by the pandemic endure; at the same time, safety net programs are being curtailed, returning at-risk populations to their prior levels of vulnerability.

The fallout of the COVID-19-induced shutdown made clear that the workers most essential to the US economy (i.e., those working in the food, health, and transportation sectors) are among the most vulnerable as well. The multisectoral spillover effects from the stay-at-home order also served as a reminder that socioeconomic policies and health policies are one and the same. Clearly, health and socioeconomic vulnerabilities in the United States are intertwined, and interactions between them need to be more forcefully recognized. Even absent a pandemic, many workers are just one major illness away from job loss and potential financial catastrophe.

Rather than returning to pre–COVID-19 levels, protecting workers requires maintaining and expanding social safety net programs that address the broader fallout of potential workplace disruption, including decoupling health care access from employment, increasing child-care and mental health support, and implementing more rigorous on-site worker protections, among others. As noted by Baker, the pandemic did not create disparities but exacerbated already existing ones. If we do not learn from this historical crisis, there is little doubt that similar inequities along these familiar lines will be revealed again in future pandemics. *AJPH*

CORRESPONDENCE

Correspondence should be sent to D. Phuong Do, PhD, 1240 N 10th St, Milwaukee, WI 53205 (e-mail: dphuong@uwm.edu). Reprints can be ordered at http://www.ajph.org by clicking the "Reprints" link.

PUBLICATION INFORMATION

Full Citation: Do DP, Frank R. The short and the long arm of the COVID-19 pandemic: direct and indirect effects of the US economic lockdown. *Am J Public Health*. 2023;113(6):612–614.

Acceptance Date: February 28, 2023.

DOI: https://doi.org/10.2105/AJPH.2023.307277

CONTRIBUTORS

D. Phuong Do framed, drafted, and revised the article. R. Frank drafted and revised the article.

ACKNOWLEDGMENTS

We thank the three anonymous reviewers, including an *AJPH* associate editor, for their helpful feedback on the initial draft of this editorial.

CONFLICTS OF INTEREST

The authors declare no conflicts of interest.

REFERENCES

1. Baker MG. Nonrelocatable occupations at increased risk during pandemics: United States, 2018. *Am J Public Health*. 2020;110(8):1126–1132. https://doi.org/10.2105/AJPH.2020.305738
2. Center on Budget and Policy Priorities. Tracking the COVID-19 economy's effects on food, housing, and employment hardships. Available at: https://www.cbpp.org/research/poverty-and-inequality/tracking-the-covid-19-economys-effects-on-food-housing-and. Accessed December 15, 2022.
3. Do DP, Frank R. US frontline workers and COVID-19 inequities. *Prev Med*. 2021;153:106833. https://doi.org/10.1016/j.ypmed.2021.106833
4. Billock R, Steege A, Miniño A. *COVID-19 Mortality by Usual Occupation and Industry: 46 States and New York City, United States, 2020*. Washington, DC: National Center for Health Statistics; 2022.
5. Centers for Disease Control and Prevention. COVID-19 provisional counts: health disparities. Available at: https://www.cdc.gov/nchs/nvss/vsrr/covid19/health_disparities.htm. Accessed October 6, 2022.
6. Matthay EC, Duchowny KA, Riley AR, et al. Occupation and educational attainment characteristics associated with COVID-19 mortality by race and ethnicity in California. *JAMA Netw Open*. 2022;5(4):e228406. https://doi.org/10.1001/jamanetworkopen.2022.8406
7. Kochhar R, Bennett J. US labor market inches back from the COVID-19 shock, but recovery is far from complete. Available at: https://www.pewresearch.org/fact-tank/2021/04/14/u-s-labor-market-inches-back-from-the-covid-19-shock-but-recovery-is-far-from-complete. Accessed December 9, 2022.
8. Coleman-Jensen A, Rabbitt MP, Gregory CA, Singh A. Household food security in the United States in 2020. Available at: https://www.ers.usda.gov/webdocs/publications/102076/err-298.pdf. Accessed October 6, 2022.
9. Carli LL. Women, gender equality and COVID-19. *Gend Manag*. 2020;35(7/8):647–655. https://doi.org/10.1108/GM-07-2020-0236
10. Piquero AR, Jennings WG, Jemison E, Kaukinen C, Knaul FM. Domestic violence during the COVID-19 pandemic—evidence from a systematic review and meta-analysis. *J Crim Justice*. 2021;74:101806. https://doi.org/10.1016/j.jcrimjus.2021.101806
11. Fairlie R. The impact of COVID-19 on small business owners: evidence from the first three months after widespread social-distancing restrictions. *J Econ Manag Strategy*. 2020;29(4):727–740. https://doi.org/10.1111/jems.12400
12. Fahle E, Kane TJ, Patterson T, Reardon SF, Staiger DO. Local achievement impacts of the pandemic. Available at: https://educationrecoveryscorecard.org/wp-content/uploads/2022/10/Education-Recovery-Scorecard_Key-Findings_102822.pdf. Accessed October 6, 2022.
13. Piacentini J, Frazis H, Meyer PB, Schultz M, Sveikauskas L. The impact of COVID-19 on labor markets and inequality. Available at: https://www.bls.gov/osmr/research-papers/2022/ec220060.htm. Accessed October 6, 2022.
14. Parolin Z, Collyer S, Curran MA. Sixth child tax credit payment kept 3.7 million children out of poverty in December. Available at: https://static1.squarespace.com/static/610831a16c95260dbd68934a/t/61ea09926280d03df62aa31d/1642727841927/Monthly-poverty-December-2021-CPSP.pdf. Accessed October 6, 2022.
15. Hamilton L, Roll S, Despard M, et al. The impacts of the 2021 expanded child tax credit on family employment, nutrition, and financial well-being. Available at: https://www.brookings.edu/research/the-impacts-of-the-2021-expanded-child-tax-credit-on-family-employment-nutrition-and-financial-well-being. Accessed December 15, 2022.

Vaccine Uptake and Hesitancy in Rural America in the Wake of the COVID-19 Pandemic

Timothy Callaghan, PhD

ABOUT THE AUTHORS

Timothy Callaghan is an associate professor in the Department of Health Law, Policy, and Management at the Boston University School of Public Health, Boston, MA.

See also Soorapanth et al., p. 680.

Since the onset of the COVID-19 pandemic, persistent disparities in the burden of disease have been seen between rural and urban areas of the United States. Despite lacking the population density in which we would expect COVID-19 to propagate most easily, rural areas have consistently had a higher incidence of COVID-19 relative to population size than urban areas.[1–3] With rural Americans more likely than their urban counterparts to be older and sicker and to hold more chronic conditions associated with poor COVID-19 outcomes, this high case incidence has had devastating consequences for many rural communities throughout the United States.[4] Rural mortality rates for COVID-19 have consistently surpassed urban mortality rates since the fall of 2020, with little reason to expect a reversal in that trend.[5,6]

While the older age and comorbidity status of rural communities do place them at higher risk for negative COVID-19 outcomes, scholars have pointed to two additional factors to explain the higher burden of COVID-19 in rural communities: limitations in health care access and lower levels of adoption of preventive health behaviors. In the area of access, almost 66% of health professional shortage areas nationwide are located in rural areas, and more than 140 rural hospitals have closed since 2010 (https://unc.live/3zaXFJC; https://bit.ly/40GzRsR). When paired with the higher travel burden that rural Americans face in accessing care, rural Americans are placed at a considerable disadvantage for positive outcomes when they become sick with COVID-19.[7]

Simultaneously, other research has pointed to differences in the adoption of preventive health behaviors across rural and urban communities in explaining differences in COVID-19 outcomes. For example, my past work suggests that rural Americans have been less likely to wear face masks than urban Americans,[8] and other research points to rural Americans also being less likely to vaccinate.[9] Combined, these behavioral differences place rural Americans at a higher risk for contracting COVID-19 and facing its severe consequences.

Despite the importance of this existing work on COVID-19 in rural America, critical questions remain. Most notably, more work is needed in the area of vaccination to understand the extent to which lower vaccine uptake in rural communities is the result of higher levels of hesitancy in rural communities or the result of the many challenges that rural Americans face in accessing primary and preventive care including vaccination.

RURAL VACCINE UPTAKE, HESITANCY, AND ACCESS

In this issue of *AJPH*, Soorapanth et al. (p. 680) begin to answer this question with one of the most comprehensive studies to date on rural versus urban vaccine uptake and hesitancy. Relying on survey data from the COVID-19 Trends and Impact Survey (CTIS) collected over Facebook from May 2021 to April 2022 and rurality information derived from zip codes and Rural–Urban Commuting Area codes, Soorapanth et al. explored the nuanced relationship between vaccination rates, vaccination hesitancy, and vaccination refusal in rural and urban communities.

In line with past research, Soorapanth et al. found that, across most states, rural areas had lower levels of COVID-19 vaccination during their period of analysis. Simultaneously, however, they found that hesitancy—which they defined as the proportion of the public who are unvaccinated but who state they probably will or will not get vaccinated—was only different between rural and urban areas in 12% of states examined. Similarly, the vaccine refusal rate—which the researchers defined as individuals who are unvaccinated and state that they definitely will not vaccinate—was only different between rural and urban areas in 21% of states examined.

The study by Soorapanth et al. adds important nuance to the literature on vaccination in rural areas that was previously missing. While vaccination rates are consistently lower in rural

AJPH June 2023, Vol 113, No. 6

areas, the difference in uptake appears to be infrequently attributable to differences in future intention to vaccinate among the unvaccinated. The major strength of the study by Soorapanth et al. is the scope of the sample they relied on. The CTIS surveyed upward of 40 000 respondents per day, over the course of the year, providing a massive sample of respondents in both rural and urban communities to study. The research also presents an intriguing idea in its discussion, suggesting that instead of hesitancy explaining the discrepancy between vaccine uptake and intentions between rural and urban communities, access issues could instead explain this difference.

With that said, there are several limitations of the study by Soorapanth et al. that should be acknowledged as well. Critically, while the authors suspected that access could explain the discrepancy between uptake and hesitancy, they provided no evidence that access explained the difference observed. It certainly *could* be the case that limited access to vaccines in rural communities has led to lower levels of uptake, but more research would be needed to support that conclusion. Three years into the COVID-19 pandemic, I find access to be a less convincing argument. While pockets of vulnerable individuals in rural America may not yet have had access to vaccination, the majority of rural Americans have had the chance to vaccinate. Exploring the potential role of access in explaining the discrepancy between uptake and hesitancy is a vital next step for the literature.

Equally important, the study did not include several covariates that could alternatively help to explain both vaccine uptake and hesitancy. The lack of a measure of partisanship is particularly glaring. The COVID-19 pandemic has seen lower levels of vaccine uptake and higher hesitancy among conservatives, driven in part by the concerted effort of antivax advocacy groups, influencers, and key Republican politicians.[10] With rural areas across the country tending to be conservative, the article by Soorapanth et al. could be missing a key determinant of vaccine uptake or hesitancy. Similarly, future rural vaccination research would benefit from the inclusion of measures of rural identity.[11] The extent to which rural Americans feel a sense of closeness with rural life and other rural Americans could shape willingness to adopt prosocial health behaviors like vaccination and also help to explain the researchers' finding that rural Americans were more likely to trust health information from friends and family.

THE FUTURE OF RURAL VACCINE HESITANCY RESEARCH

Ultimately, Soorapanth's article presents a useful jumping-off point for additional research on vaccine uptake and hesitancy in rural America in the wake of the COVID-19 pandemic. Additional research is clearly needed to untangle the discrepancy between lower uptake in rural America but not higher levels of hesitancy. Investigations of access should feature prominently into these studies, but so should investigations of political beliefs and rural identity. Just as important, additional research using other (non-CTIS) platforms provides the opportunity to innovate in survey design. Efforts should be made to capture vaccine hesitancy as the spectrum that it is instead of using a single survey item. Relatedly, capturing the full diversity and gradations of rurality instead of relying on single rural-versus-urban items would be a useful advance. Finally, moving beyond cross-sectional research to focus on changing uptake and hesitancy within individuals over time would be valuable.

Regardless of whether it is driven by access challenges, political circumstances, hesitancy, or any other factor, additional interventions are clearly needed to address the lower levels of vaccine uptake in rural communities. Without targeted efforts, rural–urban disparities in health outcomes will continue to be exacerbated by COVID-19, placing unnecessary additional burden on an already strained rural health care system. AJPH

CORRESPONDENCE

Correspondence should be sent to Timothy Callaghan, 715 Albany St, Boston, MA 02118 (e-mail: timcal@bu.edu). Reprints can be ordered at https://ajph.org by clicking the "Reprints" link.

PUBLICATION INFORMATION

Full Citation: Callaghan T. Vaccine uptake and hesitancy in rural America in the wake of the COVID-19 pandemic. *Am J Public Health*. 2023; 113(6):615–617.

Acceptance Date: March 23, 2023.

DOI: https://doi.org/10.2105/AJPH.2023.307305

CONFLICTS OF INTEREST

The author has no conflicts of interest to declare.

REFERENCES

1. Pender J. The COVID-19 pandemic and rural America. US Department of Agriculture, Economic Research Service. October 11, 2022. Available at: https://www.ers.usda.gov/covid-19/rural-america. Accessed December 4, 2022.
2. Lakhani HV, Pillai SS, Zehra M, Sharma I, Sodhi K. Systematic review of clinical insights into novel coronavirus (COVID-19) pandemic: persisting challenges in U.S. rural population. *Int J Environ Res Public Health*. 2020;17(12):4279. https://doi.org/10.3390/ijerph17124279
3. Ranscombe P. Rural areas at risk during COVID-19 pandemic. *Lancet Infect Dis*. 2020;20(5):545. https://doi.org/10.1016/S1473-3099(20)30301-7
4. Peters DJ. Community susceptibility and resiliency to COVID-19 across the rural–urban

continuum in the United States. *J Rural Health.* 2020; 36(3):446–456. https://doi.org/10.1111/jrh.12477

5. Yue S, Cheng KJG, Monnat SM. Rural–urban and within-rural differences in COVID-19 mortality rates. *J Rural Soc Sci.* 2022;37(2):article 3. Available at: https://egrove.olemiss.edu/jrss/vol37/iss2/3. Accessed March 28, 2023.
6. Dobis EA, McGranahan D. Rural death rates from COVID-19 surpassed urban death rates in early September 2020. Chart detail. US Department of Agriculture, Economic Research Service. March 19, 2021. Available at: https://www.ers.usda.gov/data-products/chart-gallery/gallery/chart-detail/?chartId=100740. Accessed December 4, 2022.
7. Akinlotan M, Primm K, Khodakarami N, Bolin J, Ferdinand A. Rural–urban variations in travel burdens for care: findings from the 2017 National Household Travel Survey. College Station, TX: Southwest Rural Health Research Center; 2021.
8. Callaghan T, Lueck JA, Trujillo KL, Ferdinand AO. Rural and urban differences in COVID-19 prevention behaviors. *J Rural Health.* 2021;37(2):287–295. https://doi.org/10.1111/jrh.12556
9. Murthy BP, Sterrett N, Weller D, et al. Disparities in COVID-19 vaccination coverage between urban and rural counties—United States, December 14, 2020–April 10, 2021. *MMWR Morb Mortal Wkly Rep.* 2021;70(20):759–764. https://doi.org/10.15585/mmwr.mm7020e3
10. Sharfstein JM, Callaghan T, Carpiano RM, et al. Uncoupling vaccination from politics: a call to action. *Lancet.* 2021;398(10307):1211–1212. https://doi.org/10.1016/S0140-6736(21)02099-7
11. Lunz Trujillo K. Rural identity as a contributing factor to anti-intellectualism in the US. *Polit Behav.* 2022;44(3):1509–1532. https://doi.org/10.1007/s11109-022-09770-w

Public Health Data of the People, by the People, for the People: A Public Health of Consequence, June 2023

Farzana Kapadia, PhD, MPH

ABOUT THE AUTHOR

Farzana Kapadia is the deputy editor of AJPH *and a professor of epidemiology at the School of Global Public Health, New York University, New York.*

See also Krieger et al., p. 667.

AJPH June 2023, Vol 113, No. 6

All public health professionals recognize the importance of ongoing, timely, and accurate surveillance and monitoring of population health as an essential foundation of our work—whether that work involves research, training, program planning, policy implementation, prevention activities, or advocacy efforts. We constantly rely on data from the many national and state-level surveillance and monitoring systems to understand population-level health and well-being and health disparities experienced by different groups of people. Importantly, we use data from these systems to understand how health and health care disparities evolve—either widening or narrowing—in the context of social, political, economic, and environmental shocks as well as in relation to policy mandates.

But what happens if one or more of these surveillance systems is not able to provide an accurate picture of population health? And what happens when these problems appear during a critical period of social, political, and economic shocks? In this issue of *AJPH*, Krieger et al. (p. 667) present information on one of these problems: the alarming decreases in response rates across six national US surveys in 2020 compared with those in 2019. In reviewing these decreasing response rates and what they could mean for understanding population health indicators, we also discuss the opportunities that this moment presents to embed principles of equity and social justice in our data collection systems. Critically, these opportunities call for novel ways of thinking about the relationships between those who use the data and those who provide the data.

SURVEYS: WHO RESPONDS, WHO DOES NOT

Given that the pandemic significantly curtailed survey operations, people who did not require multiple follow-up attempts were more likely to complete surveys than those who did. Krieger et al. review response rates for six major US surveys: three social or economic focused and three health focused. Krieger et al. appear to be the first to document how these response rates have changed between the prepandemic period (2019–February 2020) and since the onset of the pandemic (March 2020–2022). Although their findings indicate that response rates for five out of six of these national surveys decreased substantially during the pandemic, more alarming is the pattern of decrease, which paints a picture that is not an accurate reflection of the health, social, and economic status of the US population. As summarized in the survey documentation presented for the US Census American Community Survey:

> Groups that tend to be underrepresented in the estimates, such as the Black non-Hispanic and the Hispanic populations, had lower coverage rates and were less represented in 2020. . . . These data make it appear that the U.S. population had higher levels of education, had more married couples and fewer never married individuals, had less Medicaid coverage, had higher median household incomes, had fewer noncitizens, and were more likely to live in single-family housing units. In the midst of a pandemic that negatively affected so many lives in 2020, these data show that the respondents were not nationally representative and that the weighting methods did not account for the non-response bias. (https://bit.ly/3mYhfG9)

Across these survey systems, working with community-based partners has been a cornerstone to obtaining robust response rates. Moving forward, it remains to be seen whether these trends in nonresponse will continue once survey teams across these programs are fully operational and deployed to reach representative samples across our population.

Equally important is the application of an equity-focused lens to ensure that the data collected reflect our collective goal of social justice.

DATA COLLECTION FOR DATA EQUITY

The impact of the COVID-19 pandemic on response rates, as summarized by Krieger et al., provides a compelling call for revitalizing US public health data collection systems to incorporate social justice and equity measures throughout the life cycle of data collection. Several efforts are under way, reflecting the immediacy of these concerns and the need to rapidly translate these recommendations into practice.

The Urban Institute has issued a set of guidelines that "frame ways to make affected communities and groups of people a first-tier consideration throughout the data life cycle" (https://urbn.is/3JRKrrk). The guideline employs the Belmont Report's tenets of beneficence, respect for persons, and justice to data practice at all levels, including conceptualization, instrumentation (measurement), collection, processing and analysis, and dissemination. These guidelines provide a framework for community inclusion in decision-making on which data are to be collected, transparency in how the data are collected and among whom, and how the data are used and disseminated—all with an eye to how data collection activities and publication may reinforce or reduce inequities.

In October 2021, the Robert Wood Johnson Foundation launched the National Commission to Transform Public Health Data Systems to "reimagine how data are collected, shared, and used, and identify the investments needed to improve health equity" (http://bit.ly/3lPSNqj). This is yet another investment signaling the need to work across sectors and to conscientiously, carefully, and creatively work with communities to ensure data equity via the collection of information requisite to promote health equity and social justice.

Finally, the Centers for Disease Control and Prevention Foundation has issued the report "Principles for Using Public Health Data to Drive Equity" (https://bit.ly/3ZlQEjK), which reinforces the call for greater community inclusion and a focus on community-level change that can help fell the structural racism and discrimination that drive health inequities.

This is a moment when we see how the shortcomings in our national- and state-level data collection can be mitigated. This moment also presents the opportunity for fostering systems that are more inclusive and for obtaining the data we need to promote population health and strive toward a public health of consequence. AJPH

CORRESPONDENCE

Correspondence should be sent to Farzana Kapadia, PhD, MPH, New York University, School of Global Public Health, 708 Broadway, Room 729, New York, NY 10003 (e-mail: farzana.kapadia@nyu.edu). Reprints can be ordered at http://www.ajph.org by clicking the "Reprints" link.

PUBLICATION INFORMATION

Full Citation: Kapadia F. Public health data of the people, by the people, for the people: a public health of consequence, June 2023. *Am J Public Health*. 2023;113(6):618–619.

Acceptance Date: March 19, 2023.

DOI: https://doi.org/10.2105/AJPH.2023.307295

CONFLICTS OF INTEREST

The author has no conflicts of interest to disclose.

Addressing the Need for Accountability in Public Health

Sonja A. Rasmussen, MD, MS, Richard A. Goodman, MD, JD, MPH, and Wendy E. Parmet, JD

ABOUT THE AUTHORS

Sonja A. Rasmussen is with the Johns Hopkins University School of Medicine, Baltimore, MD. Richard A. Goodman is with the Department of Family and Preventive Medicine, Emory University School of Medicine, Atlanta, GA. Wendy E. Parmet is with the Center for Health Policy and Law, Northeastern University School of Law, Boston, MA.

AJPH June 2023, Vol 113, No. 6

The proliferation of information contrary to scientific evidence has undermined efforts to control the COVID-19 pandemic. Most public health officials have worked valiantly to provide scientifically grounded recommendations and other information to the public on issues such as social distancing, vaccines, and masking. However, a few have issued statements or offered guidance departing from the best available evidence.[1,2] Such statements can contribute to confusion, disregard for and rejection of science-based guidance, and mistrust of the public health system. They may be especially problematic because individuals seeking to keep themselves and their families healthy may rely on the recommendations of public officials who purportedly have expertise about public health.

The dissemination of advice that is not supported by science can also undermine the public's trust in public health officials, jeopardizing public health's capacity to protect health moving forward. Here we call for the public health community to examine how to deter the issuance of deficiently supported recommendations by holding accountable public health officials who promote such recommendations.

ADVICE THAT CONTRADICTS THE EVIDENCE

As an example of public health advice that contradicts prevailing scientific evidence, Florida's surgeon general, a licensed physician appointed by the Florida governor in 2021 to serve as the secretary of health for the Florida Department of Health, announced on March 7, 2022, that Florida would be the first state to officially recommend against COVID-19 vaccines for healthy children. This statement conflicted with recommendations from the Centers for Disease Control and Prevention (and its independent advisory committee, the Advisory Committee on Immunization Practices) and the American Academy of Pediatrics; notably, we are not aware of any other states that have followed suit.

More recently, the Florida surgeon general recommended against administration of mRNA COVID-19 vaccines for men 18 to 39 years of age, apparently on the basis of a single non–peer-reviewed analysis by the Florida Department of Health published online without named authors. As with the previous recommendation, experts and professional organizations vigorously denounced this statement.[3,4] Despite that criticism, the Florida Department of Health reiterated these recommendations on December 2, 2022, with a provider alert stating that "based on the currently available data, Florida's Surgeon General does not recommend the COVID-19 vaccines for healthy children and adolescents or the mRNA vaccines for males ages 18 to 39 because the risks likely outweigh the benefits at this point in the pandemic."[5]

Dissemination of recommendations that conflict with scientific evidence by public health officials—individuals who are responsible for the health of a jurisdiction on the basis of their position, whether they are political appointees or government civil servants—can lead people to act in ways that jeopardize their health and that of their families and communities. Undermining confidence in the safety and effectiveness of COVID-19 vaccines has the potential to further undermine the public's trust in other vaccines, already a significant concern as seen recently with declining public support for childhood vaccine mandates,[6] which places one of public health's top achievements[7] at risk.

In addition, guidance not based on scientific evidence can erode the public's trust in public health. As stated in the American Public Health Association's Code of Ethics, "The effectiveness of public health policies, practices, and actions depends upon public trust gained through decisions based on the highest ethical, scientific, and professional standards. Public health gains public trust in part because its practices are informed by evidence." The code, however, was developed as guidance and is not enforceable; indeed, it specifically states that "it is not intended to be used to discipline and sanction professional misconduct."[8]

MECHANISMS FOR ACCOUNTABILITY

It is time for public health to rethink the question of whether and how the profession can hold to account health officials who offer information that departs from scientific evidence as it exists at the time the advice is offered. Although many public health officials (e.g., physicians and nurses) are licensed health care professionals, not all are, and states do not license public health workers as a specific category. Nevertheless, mechanisms developed to hold physicians accountable might be applied to public health professionals.

In an article on physicians whose actions threatened the nation's health during the COVID-19 pandemic, Pizzo et al.[9] listed professional self-regulation through state licensing boards, professional certification, or professional societies as an important mechanism for accountability when physicians violate their ethical responsibilities. Such an approach may be applicable to public health officials who are licensed health care professionals but cannot be applied to those who are not. However, Pizzo et al.[9] pointed to another mechanism for accountability: professional organizations can be influential by stating that the physician's actions violate professional conduct standards. This approach, as applied to public health officials, holds potential for minimizing adverse effects on the public's health even in the absence of sanctions. Although professional societies can provide a voice highlighting when recommendations run counter to scientific evidence, it is unlikely that these pronouncements will be sufficient to hold rogue officials accountable.

Pizzo et al.[9] discussed another mechanism for accountability among physicians (that may also be relevant to health professionals other than physicians) that applies specifically to those who are affiliated with a university. University and other academic institution leaders can publicly state that the institution does not endorse the actions of a faculty member when they are contrary to scientific evidence.

For example, when Dr. Scott Atlas, a neuroradiologist, provided guidance to the White House early in the pandemic that conflicted with the prevailing science, Stanford University, with which he was affiliated, issued the following statement: "Dr. Atlas has expressed views that are inconsistent with the university's approach in response to the pandemic. Dr. Atlas's statements reflect his personal views, not those of the Hoover Institution or the university."[10] However, Pizzo et al.[9] also noted that issues of academic freedom might complicate this response and that university faculty members can express their disapproval, as seen at Stanford. The Stanford faculty senate adopted a resolution strongly condemning Dr. Atlas's actions, stating that his actions "promote a view of COVID-19 that contradicts medical science."[10,11]

In a prepandemic article on accountability in health care, Emanuel and Emanuel[12] discussed the potential role of economic incentives in policing health care providers. They noted, for example, that patients may switch physicians who fail to conform to professional standards. Although this is an option for an individual patient who is dissatisfied with a physician's care, it is not an option in public health: residents of a state, county, or other local jurisdiction served by a public health official who fails to follow scientific guidance cannot simply choose another public health official. Moreover, even if some residents opt to ignore the erroneous advice, they may face increased risks if others in their community do not (e.g., by forgoing vaccination). Waiting for the next election to change the administration that selected the public health official is an option, but health can be endangered in the interim. Furthermore, voters elect officials on the basis of a wide variety of issues including, but not limited to, public health.

Another mechanism for professional accountability listed by Emanuel and Emanuel[12] is medical malpractice. Dissemination of statements that contradict scientific evidence by public health officials bears striking similarity to medical malpractice, which encompasses the provision of advice that departs from the standard of care in medicine. If a medical malpractice claim is to be successful, a plaintiff must show that the defendant owed the plaintiff a duty of care, that the defendant breached that duty by failing to act in accordance with the standard of care, and that the breach was the factual and legal cause of the plaintiff's injuries. Medical practitioners are expected to practice to the standard of a reasonable practitioner under the circumstances (customary practice).[13] Failure to conform to this standard can lead to legal liability and, more rarely, can result in disciplinary actions by licensing boards.

Although a legal claim for "public health malpractice" as such has not been recognized by the courts, researchers have explored the idea of treating the dissemination of false and erroneous misinformation by health officials as a form of public health malpractice. For example, Parmet and Haupt discussed the similarities between the dissemination by physicians of medical advice that departs from professional standards, which the law of malpractice polices, and the provision of advice that departs from professional standards by health officials.[14,15] As they explained it, the professional in both cases has a fiduciary obligation to the recipient (individual patient or the public) of the "bad advice" who may be harmed by the advice. Although Parmet and Haupt found the similarities between medical malpractice and public health malpractice compelling, they also noted that there are substantial legal barriers to the adjudication of claims against public officials, including but not limited to legal immunities for public officials.

Claims of "public health malpractice" might be one option for accountability among public health officials, but this would take the issue of accountability out of the hands of public health professionals and into the courts. Such a move could be potentially risky because courts might not be well suited to judge whether advice departs from community standards. In addition, public health officials might be required to respond to "nuisance" claims, consuming time needed for responding to a public health emergency.

NEED FOR SELF-REGULATION

Ensuring accountability for public health officials raises a host of issues, such as what types of missteps would trigger the need for accountability. We propose that accountability be focused on the most egregious recommendations that clearly contradict scientific evidence. Despite the challenges, other professions (e.g., physicians, dentists, nurses, lawyers) have developed mechanisms, although imperfect, to hold their members responsible for meeting professional standards. We believe that the public health community as a profession needs to explore options and develop solutions for accountability among its members. Self-regulation is a traditional attribute of professions, and accountability from within the field might help to ward off other forms of sanctions from the courts or in the political sphere that would take the role out of the hands of public health experts.

Most public health officials have worked heroically over the past few years, often under very trying conditions. Efforts to address the need for accountability among public health officials should be designed so as not to burden them but to provide a path for holding accountable the very few who depart from customary practice and endanger the public's health. Such accountability may be critical to ensuring that the public does not receive and rely on dangerous public health advice in the future. It may also facilitate the work of the majority of health officials whose efforts depend on securing the public's trust. AJPH

CORRESPONDENCE

Correspondence should be sent to Sonja A. Rasmussen, MD, MS, 600 N Wolfe St, Blalock 1007, Baltimore, MD 21287 (e-mail: srasmus2@jhu.edu). Reprints can be ordered at http://www.ajph.org by clicking the "Reprints" link.

PUBLICATION INFORMATION

Full Citation: Rasmussen SA, Goodman RA, Parmet WE. Addressing the need for accountability in public health. *Am J Public Health*. 2023;113(6):620–622.

Acceptance Date: March 13, 2023.

DOI: https://doi.org/10.2105/AJPH.2023.307290

CONTRIBUTORS

The authors contributed equally to this work.

CONFLICTS OF INTEREST

The authors have no conflicts of interest to declare.

REFERENCES

1. Rubin R. When physicians spread unscientific information about COVID-19. *JAMA*. 2022;327(10):904–906. https://doi.org/10.1001/jama.2022.1083
2. Goodman CK, Catherman C. CDC, FDA send letter to Florida's surgeon general warning he is endangering lives with COVID vaccine risk advice. Available at: https://www.sun-sentinel.com/health/fl-ne-letter-to-florida-surgeon-general-20230310-ni3gmpvf6bertmozhghdcqungu-story.html. Accessed March 12, 2023.
3. Flaherty A. Scientists pan analysis Florida's surgeon general posted on COVID-19 vaccines. Available at: https://abcnews.go.com/Health/scientists-pan-analysis-floridas-surgeon-general-posted-covid/story?id=91294952. Accessed January 22, 2022.
4. Diamond D. Experts slam Florida surgeon general's warning on coronavirus vaccines. Available at: https://www.washingtonpost.com/health/2022/10/11/florida-surgeon-general-ladapo-covid-vaccines. Accessed March 8, 2023.
5. Florida Department of Health. Provider alert: COVID-19 boosters. Available at: https://www.floridahealth.gov/newsroom/2022/12/20221202-provider-alert-covid19-boosters.pr.html. Accessed December 17, 2022.
6. Lopes L, Schumacher S, Sparks G, Presiado M, Hamel L, Brodie M. KFF COVID-19 Vaccine Monitor: December 2022. Available at: https://www.kff.org/coronavirus-covid-19/poll-finding/kff-covid-19-vaccine-monitor-december-2022. Accessed January 22, 2023.
7. Centers for Disease Control and Prevention. Ten great public health achievements—worldwide, 2001–2010. *MMWR Morb Mortal Wkly Rep*. 2011;60(24):814–818.
8. American Public Health Association. Public Health Code of Ethics (2019 version). Available at: https://www.apha.org/-/media/files/pdf/membergroups/ethics/code_of_ethics.ashx. Accessed January 22, 2023.
9. Pizzo PA, Spiegel D, Mello MM. When physicians engage in practices that threaten the nation's health. *JAMA*. 2021;325(8):723–724. https://doi.org/10.1001/jama.2021.0122
10. Nietzel MT. Stanford faculty senate condemns Dr. Scott Atlas over his COVID-19 conduct. Available at: https://www.forbes.com/sites/michaeltnietzel/2020/11/21/stanford-faculty-senate-condems-dr-scott-atlas-over-his-covid-19-conduct/?sh=6a49f08d685e. Accessed January 22, 2023.
11. Chesley K. Faculty senate condemns COVID-19 actions of Hoover's Scott Atlas. Available at: https://news.stanford.edu/2020/11/20/faculty-senate-condemns-actions-hoover-fellow-scott-atlas. Accessed January 24, 2023.
12. Emanuel EJ, Emanuel LL. What is accountability in health care? *Ann Intern Med*. 1996;124(2):229–239. https://doi.org/10.7326/0003-4819-124-2-199601150-00007
13. Studdert DM, Hall MA. Medical malpractice law—doctrine and dynamics. *N Engl J Med*. 2022;387(17):1533–1537. https://doi.org/10.1056/NEJMp2201675
14. Parmet WE, Haupt CE. Holding clinicians in public office accountable to professional standards. *AMA J Ethics*. 2023;25(3):E194–E199. https://doi.org/10.1001/amajethics.2023.194
15. Haupt CE, Parmet WE. Lethal lies: government speech, distorted science, and the First Amendment. *Univ Ill Law Rev*. 2022;2022:1809–1844.

Public Libraries for Public Health: COVID-19 Response Efforts in Prince George's County, Maryland

Diego de Acosta, PhD, Nicholas Alexander Brown, MSLIS, Rachel Zukowski, MEd, Erin Mann, MPH, and Elizabeth Dawson-Hahn, MD, MPH

Public libraries—trusted institutions with broad population reach—are well positioned to partner with public health departments to advance community health. In 2020 through 2022, Prince George's County Memorial Library System assumed increasing responsibility in the local COVID-19 pandemic response by providing information and expanded services to county residents. With additional private funding, staffing, and public health resources, this library system codeveloped interventions to address information gaps, improve language access, and connect residents to more than 120 500 KN95 masks, more than 124 300 self-test kits, and more than 2400 vaccines. (*Am J Public Health*. 2023;113(6):623–626. https://doi.org/10.2105/AJPH.2023.307246)

AJPH June 2023, Vol 113, No. 6

Public libraries are seldom recognized as public health resources, but they offer programs that address social determinants of health and regularly partner with government agencies and community organizations to facilitate access to health services and programs.[1,2] Public libraries are free, accessible, and widely trusted institutions with significant population reach. In a 2016 Pew Research Center survey, 78% of adults said public libraries help them find trustworthy, reliable information.[3] Approximately 316 million Americans—97% of the population—live in an area served by a public library.[4] Therefore, public libraries are well positioned to relay vital health information and host some complementary services.

INTERVENTION AND IMPLEMENTATION

Prince George's County Memorial Library System (PGCMLS), a public library network in Maryland, expanded its public health role during the COVID-19 pandemic to meet community needs and requests from the Prince George's County Health Department (PGCHD). Between spring 2020 and summer 2022, PGCMLS assumed increasing responsibility in the local COVID-19 response by providing information, aid, and expanded services to county residents (Table 1). Because the crisis developed unpredictably, PGCMLS's interventions emerged stepwise based on regular assessments.

Before March 2020, PGCMLS was offering health and wellness programming (e.g., dental screenings and yoga) and partnering with health care exchange agencies to facilitate enrollment in health coverage. At the pandemic's start, PGCMLS became one of several county organizations that published COVID-19 emergency updates. PGCMLS leveraged its role as a trusted community organization, publishing accurate information rapidly through multiple channels: the library's Web site, social media, and flyers in curbside pickup bags.

PGCMLS also participated in relief efforts such as distributing food and facilitating access to affordable health care coverage during the COVID-19 special enrollment period (the facilitated access continued pre-COVID work).

In early 2021, PGCMLS and its partners became aware of challenges to booking vaccine appointments. Capital One Foundation, a corporate philanthropy partner, offered funding and asked PGCMLS to propose a program addressing vaccine inequity. PGCMLS created the Vaccine Hunter Hotline based on crowdsourced vaccine-hunting groups on social media. The hotline launched on April 1 and initially helped county residents to access accurate vaccine information, book appointments, or preregister. Hotline operators—library staff and 11 new

TABLE 1— Timeline of Prince George's County Memorial Library System (PGCMLS) COVID-19–Related Work: Prince George's County, Maryland

2019	2020	2021	2022
(Pre-COVID) PGCMLS's 2019–2020 strategic framework identifies Healthy Living as 1 of 5 focus areas, aligning with a county government focus on healthy communities. The library system's health and wellness offerings include dental screening clinics, flu vaccine clinics, and yoga classes. These activities crucially lay the foundation for PGCMLS's interventions and public health partnership over the next 2 years.	Throughout the year, PGCMLS disseminates COVID-19 emergency public health communications and collaborates in the County Joint Information Center, supporting emergency operations. The library system offers mobile food pantry distributions, summer meals for K-12 students and, in the winter, coats for children. Health and wellness programs continue virtually.	In the spring, PGCMLS launches the Vaccine Hunter Hotline, which operates for 8½ weeks. The hotline helps more than 1240 community members with limited digital access, limited digital literacy, or limited English to navigate vaccine appointment systems. In its final phase, the hotline becomes an outreach operation, calling more than 52 170 county residents to offer information and assistance with vaccine appointments. In late fall and winter, 25 vaccine clinics are hosted at PGCMLS libraries and library-linked community events. The library system also hosts 2 winter health fairs and gives away more coats for children.	The winter vaccine clinics continue, and PGCMLS distributes more than 124 300 COVID-19 self-test kits and more than 120 500 KN95 masks. In the spring, the library system runs a Period Action Drive, collecting pads and tampons to benefit a local women's shelter. In the summer, PGCMLS launches the Community Health Worker in the Library program, focused on zip codes with high health disparities. The library system also gives away free dental health kits and shoes for children. PGCMLS replaces its COVID-19 Web page with a broader public health Web page containing resources and information about COVID-19, monkeypox, HIV, and influenza.

Note. K-12 = kindergarten through grade 12.

part-time employees—assisted callers with limited digital access or digital literacy as well as Spanish-speaking callers unable to navigate the booking system in English.

When the hotline launched, Maryland's vaccines were limited to adults aged 65 years and older, adults aged 16 to 64 years at increased risk of severe illness, health workers, and public-facing essential workers. The hotline's initial funding—$12 500—covered six weeks, but because call volumes remained high the PGCMLS Foundation added $5000 to sustain staffing.

By mid-May 2021, COVID-19 vaccines had become more plentiful: the Federal Emergency Management Agency opened walk-up sites and retail pharmacies had some overstock. The hotline's call volumes abruptly decreased. However, in a countywide forum facilitated by the PGCHD, PGCMLS staff learned of a pressing need to reach zip codes with lower vaccination rates. PGCMLS quickly converted its hotline into an outreach operation, calling residents to offer information and assistance booking vaccine appointments. In all, the Vaccine Hunter Hotline program lasted 59 business days.

Support for the hotline was as follows:

- $12 500 from Capital One Foundation to launch the program: $11 280 for the wages of 11 part-time contract staff, $720 for a social media vaccine awareness campaign, and $500 for vaccine awareness programs;
- $5000 from the PGCMLS Foundation, entirely for staffing, to support extending the program to June 2021; and
- in-kind staffing support from PGCMLS.

From September 2021 to February 2022, PGCMLS hosted 25 vaccine clinics using two models: adding clinics to scheduled library events (e.g., Hispanic Heritage Celebrations) and hosting stand-alone clinics coordinated through the PGCHD, the Maryland Department of Health, and the Maryland Vaccine Equity Task Force.

From November 2021 to May 2022, PGCMLS distributed KN95 masks and, from January to May 2022, self-test kits. This distribution drive was largely in response to community demand. During the Omicron wave in early December, Prince George's County was distributing fewer test kits but seeing higher infection rates than neighboring counties. The PGCHD approached PGCMLS and other agencies, arranging to supply kits for these agencies to distribute widely. Eventually, the urgent demand for test kits and masks waned and the distribution concluded.

PLACE, TIME, AND PERSONS

PGCMLS operates 19 branches across urban, suburban, and rural settings in

Maryland. It serves a population of 967 201 county residents, 62% of whom are Black, 21% Hispanic, 14% non-Hispanic White, and 4% Asian; 17% of county residents speak Spanish at home and 15% of county households earn less than $35 000 a year.[5] The county has traditionally relied on grassroots efforts for short-term relief during health and socioeconomic crises. PGCMLS itself has a decades-long history of offering nontraditional services and partnering with health and social service providers to improve access to resources.

PURPOSE

PGCMLS's pandemic response interventions were intended to connect county residents to emergency resources and help the local public health department (the PGCHD) implement its COVID-19 prevention and mitigation measures.

EVALUATION AND ADVERSE EFFECTS

PGCMLS collected data about items distributed, interactions with community members, and, for the Vaccine Hunter Hotline, demographic data required to book appointments.

Highlights of PGCMLS's impact include the following:

- PGCMLS and county partners helped to enroll 66% of county residents eligible for Affordable Care Act coverage.
- The Vaccine Hunter Hotline helped more than 1240 county residents to secure a vaccine. More than 2400 vaccines resulted from the hotline and the 25 vaccine clinics. During the outreach phase, staff called more than 52 170 residents.
- Most residents who secured a vaccine through the hotline (Figure 1) were Black (44%) or Hispanic (33%). By the end of August 2021, over 77% of eligible residents had received at least one dose, including over 70% of eligible Hispanic residents.[6]
- PGCMLS distributed more than 120 500 KN95 masks and more than 124 300 self-test kits.

PGCMLS's interventions led to no known adverse effects or unintended consequences for county residents. However, PGCMLS staff did experience strain in reconciling the demands of new public health work with regular library activities.

SUSTAINABILITY

The PGCHD repeatedly approached PGCMLS to help with the county's pandemic response because PGCMLS demonstrated it could connect county residents to services. With increased private funding, staffing, and access to public health resources, PGCMLS successfully expanded its public health role.

As in all partnerships, the PGCHD and PGCMLS learned from each other what was feasible given their constraints. For example, the vaccine clinics were run as a system-wide program, but it was a major strain on PGCMLS, already short-staffed, to manage so many clinic sites. Mobilizing staff to do extensive public health work drew them away from core library functions. When test kit distribution began, PGCMLS offered kits at five key branches rather than reattempting a system-wide program. Other agencies

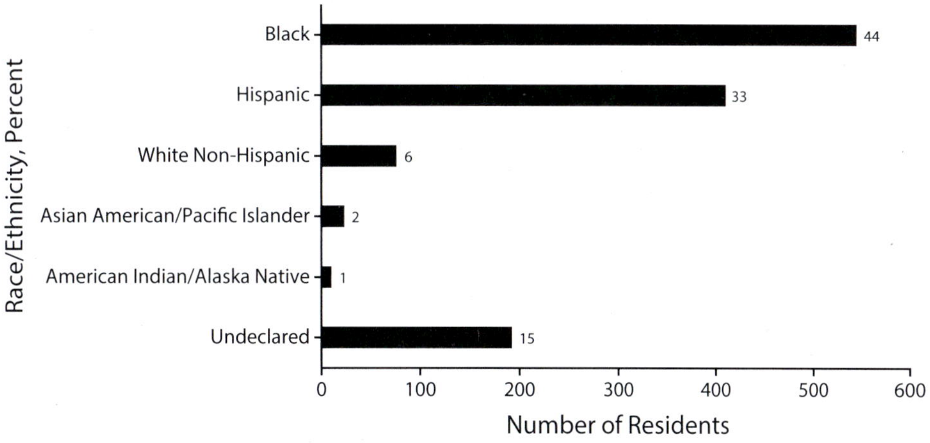

FIGURE 1— Number of County Residents Who Got a Vaccine Appointment Through the Vaccine Hunter Hotline: Prince George's County, Maryland, April–June 2021

Note. The sample size was 1245.

distributed kits at complementary sites to reach the county's whole population.

Although PGCMLS's scope of work required negotiation, the partnership between public health and libraries is thriving in Prince George's County. Thus, when the PGCHD received American Rescue Plan funding for preventative health assessments, it approached PGCMLS about starting a program that incentivized assessments with free groceries. In May 2022, PGCMLS introduced Community Health Worker in the Library, which offered public health assessments and groceries at branch libraries in areas with high health disparities.

PUBLIC HEALTH SIGNIFICANCE

The Public Health 3.0 framework calls for multisector collaboration, led by local public health departments, to advance community health and health equity.[7] PGCMLS's pandemic response suggests that public libraries can play an important role as public health partners.

PGCMLS's crisis work in 2020 through 2022 recalls the way public libraries pivoted to serve as information hubs and distribution points after recent natural disasters in the South and Midwest.[8] But although libraries' ability to pivot in crises is impressive, their strength is their dependability as trusted institutions that connect people to information and services. Public library and public health partnerships can effectively address the information divides that contribute to health disparities during both crises and normal times.[9] AJPH

ABOUT THE AUTHORS

Diego de Acosta and Erin Mann are with the National Resource Center for Refugees, Immigrants, and Migrants (NRC-RIM), University of Minnesota, Minneapolis. Nicholas Alexander Brown and Rachel Zukowski are with Prince George's County Memorial Library System, Largo, MD. Elizabeth Dawson-Hahn is with NRC-RIM, University of Minnesota, Minneapolis, and the Department of Pediatrics, University of Washington, Seattle.

CORRESPONDENCE

Correspondence should be sent to Diego de Acosta, PhD, Mayo Bldg, Suite C311, 420 Delaware St SE, Minneapolis, MN 55455 (e-mail: deaco011@umn.edu). Reprints can be ordered at http://www.ajph.org by clicking the "Reprints" link.

PUBLICATION INFORMATION

Full Citation: de Acosta D, Brown NA, Zukowski R, Mann E, Dawson-Hahn E. Public libraries for public health: COVID-19 response efforts in Prince George's County, Maryland. *Am J Public Health*. 2023;113(6):623–626.

Acceptance Date: January 22, 2023.

DOI: https://doi.org/10.2105/AJPH.2023.307246

CONTRIBUTORS

D. de Acosta led the writing and analyses. N. A. Brown and R. Zukowski co-coordinated the interventions and data gathering and assisted with the writing. E. Mann assisted with the writing and conceptualization of the study. E. Dawson-Hahn was team lead and assisted with the writing.

ACKNOWLEDGMENTS

This work was performed under the National Resource Center for Refugees, Immigrants, and Migrants (NRC-RIM), which is funded by the US Centers for Disease Control and Prevention and the International Organization for Migration (award no. CK000495-03-00/ES1874). The Prince George's County Memorial Library System (PGCMLS) health equity work was funded by Capital One Foundation and the PGCMLS Foundation.

We thank Kate Yun, MD, MS, for her review and guidance of this case study, and the members of the Qualitative Collaborative at NRC-RIM. We also acknowledge the contributions and participation of PGCMLS customers and staff.

CONFLICTS OF INTEREST

The authors have no conflicts of interest to declare.

HUMAN PARTICIPANT PROTECTION

Institutional review board approval was not needed for this study because the data used were all publicly available or obtained in aggregate.

REFERENCES

1. Philbin MM, Parker CM, Flaherty MG, Hirsch JS. Public libraries: a community-level resource to advance population health. *J Community Health*. 2019;44(1):192–199. https://doi.org/10.1007%2Fs10900-018-0547-4
2. Whiteman ED, Dupuis R, Morgan AU, et al. Public libraries as partners for health. *Prev Chronic Dis*. 2018;15:E64. 10.5888/pcd15.170392
3. Geiger AW. Most Americans—especially millennials—say libraries can help them find reliable, trustworthy information. Pew Research Center. Available at: https://www.pewresearch.org/fact-tank/2017/08/30/most-americans-especially-millennials-say-libraries-can-help-them-find-reliable-trustworthy-information. Accessed July 13, 2022.
4. Pelczar M, Frehill LM, Nielsen E, Kaiser A, Hudson J, Wan T. *Characteristics of Public Libraries in the United States: Results From the FY 2019 Public Libraries Survey*. Washington, DC: Institute of Museum and Library Services; 2021.
5. Prince George's County Health Department. Demographics: County: Prince George's. Available at: https://www.pgchealthzone.org/demographicdata?id=1260. Accessed July 28, 2022.
6. Prince George's County Executive. COVID-19 vaccine bulletin. Prince George's County Maryland. Available at: https://content.govdelivery.com/accounts/MDPGC/bulletins/2efb936. Accessed September 13, 2022.
7. DeSalvo KB, Wang YC, Harris A, Auerbach J, Koo D, O'Carroll P. Public health 3.0: a call to action for public health to meet the challenges of the 21st century. *Prev Chronic Dis*. 2017;14:E78. http://dx.doi.org/10.5888/pcd14.170017
8. Bishop B, Veil Shari R. Public libraries as post-crisis information hubs. *Public Libr Q*. 2013;32(1):33–45. https://doi.org/10.1080/01616846.2013.760390
9. Simon MA, O'Brian CA, Nava M, et al. Public libraries as key partners for advancing health equity. *Am J Public Health*. 2021;111(1):40–42. https://doi.org/10.2105/AJPH.2020.306004

The Chelsea Project: Turning Research and Wastewater Surveillance on COVID-19 Into Health Equity Action, Massachusetts, 2020–2021

Cristina Alonso, DrPH, MPH, CPM, Barry Keppard, AICP, Samantha Bates, MA, Dan Cortez, Flor Amaya, PT-DPT, MPH, and Karthik Dinakar, PhD

Chelsea, Massachusetts, had one of the highest COVID-19 transmission rates in New England in the summer of 2020. The Chelsea Project was a collaborative effort in which government entities, local nonprofit organizations, and startups partnered to deploy wastewater analysis, targeted polymerase chain reaction testing and vaccine outreach, and a community-led communications strategy. The strategy helped increase both testing rates and vaccination rates in Chelsea. Today Chelsea has one of the highest vaccination rates among US cities with comparable demographics. (*Am J Public Health.* 2023;113(6):627–630. https://doi.org/10.2105/AJPH.2023.307253)

The Center of Complex Interventions sought to create an initiative in Chelsea, Massachusetts, to build block-level sensing and intervention in response to COVID-19 in collaboration with community-based organizations (CBOs) and the city government. Leaders of the initiative, labeled the Chelsea Project (TCP), designed a system to collect and analyze data on COVID-19 rates in wastewater and collaborated with community health workers to distribute information, offer personal protective equipment, and provide vaccine appointments to residents in high-risk areas within a one-week period. This intervention demonstrates how transforming data into community action through trusted messengers has a positive impact on protective behaviors and vaccination rates.

INTERVENTION AND IMPLEMENTATION

Community survey results revealed that, as of October 2020, most people in Chelsea had not had a COVID-19 test.[1] As a response, TCP combined surveillance of virus concentrations in local wastewater, culturally resonant outreach on protective behaviors, and qualitative data from health care worker conversations held with community members. Both mobile and static testing and vaccine units responded to wastewater mapping and guidance from community health workers to determine the best locations and timing for outreach.

Wastewater Testing

Wastewater surveillance captures changes in virus concentrations, reflecting the magnitude of community transmission while ensuring anonymity. TCP collected 24-hour composite wastewater samples from four sites (selected according to population density and viability of collection) on Mondays and interpreted and communicated results through city channels.

Community-Based Organizations

Local CBOs and the Chelsea Department of Public Health received wastewater results each Wednesday afternoon. Public health directors from two CBOs and the city's communications director met every Thursday morning to discuss trends in wastewater results and vaccine rates. Communication strategies and outreach coordination were determined on the basis of these trends.

AJPH June 2023, Vol 113, No. 6

Promotoras de Salud

Two CBOs and the city department of public health hired and trained local women as community health workers (*promotoras de salud*). The *promotoras* met with one of the CBO public health directors on Thursday afternoons to report on residents' concerns regarding COVID-19, vaccines, and access to social protections. The director trained *promotoras* on the significance of recent wastewater trends and codesigned an outreach approach for that week. From Friday to Sunday, the *promotoras* targeted high-risk neighborhoods and supported residents in accessing vaccine clinics. They also spoke to residents about their concerns with COVID-19, vaccines, and other issues related to their current stressors. Through these conversations, *promotoras* were able to clarify misinformation and encourage vaccination.

Mobile Vaccine and Testing Van

TCP worked with Mass General Brigham Hospital to deploy its mobile testing and vaccine unit to high-risk neighborhoods. *Promotoras* were consulted about the best location and schedule for this van to ensure high traffic and accessibility.

Social Media

CBOs and the city provided daily updates through Facebook and TikTok on testing and vaccination and to clarify misinformation. TCP produced a series of videos with local leaders urging residents to get vaccinated. Through weekly Facebook live sessions facilitated by a CBO with a physician or public health official, residents texted their questions and received immediate answers.

Grassroots Vaccine Appointment System

Promotoras had direct access to vaccine appointments at local vaccine sites through WhatsApp. This system eliminated barriers related to accessing Web sites in English, waiting for an operator to provide an appointment, or missing confirmation callbacks.

Planning and Strategizing

TCP core members (Table 1) met every Friday to discuss weekly activities, plan for the following week, and strategize in response to citywide data and national trends.

PLACE, TIME, AND PERSONS

Chelsea occupies two square miles north of Boston. It has an estimated population of 40 000 residents, but there may be up to 75 000 residents according to informal estimates.[2] A city of mostly low-wage Latinx immigrants, it is known for having overcrowded and substandard housing and high levels of poverty and food insecurity. A study carried out in April 2020 revealed antibodies to COVID-19 among 30% of Chelsea residents.[3] By June 10, 2020, Chelsea had recorded 2839 cumulative cases of COVID-19, a rate of 7537 per 100 000, and a positivity rate of 38% (in contrast to the state positivity rate of 15%), indicating both high rates of disease and low rates of testing.[4,5] An in-depth positivity analysis showed that

TABLE 1— Names and Roles of Chelsea Project Participants: Chelsea, MA, 2021

Organization Name	Title of Participant(s)	Role in TCP
Center of Complex Interventions	Executive director Special projects director	Leadership of TCP Friday meetings Provision of funding for *promotoras*, video series, and wastewater testing
Chelsea Police Department	Community engagement specialist	Assistance in partnership building within and outside of Chelsea
City of Chelsea	Public health director Director of communications	Recruitment of *promotoras* Operation of vaccine clinic Distribution of test kits to CBOs
Metropolitan Area Planning Council	Public health director	Wastewater data analysis Vaccine data visualization
La Colaborativa	Health equity and public health director	COVID-19 positivity analysis and qualitative research Recruitment and training of *promotoras* Housing of vaccine clinic and mobile clinics Facilitation of Thursday meetings
Greenroots	Health equity and public health director	Recruitment and training of *promotoras*

Note. CBO = community-based organization; *promotoras* = *promotoras de salud* (community health workers); TCP = the Chelsea Project.

residents testing positive were mostly those who were in their 40s during the first surge of COVID-19 in summer 2020.[1]

We began wastewater testing in November 2020 and outreach efforts in January 2021. Vaccine rollout began in February 2021.

PURPOSE

TCP aimed to decrease the rates and impact of COVID-19 in Chelsea. The project design ensured that outreach, testing, and vaccine scheduling were available outside of working hours. Training and deploying *promotoras* ensured that messengers were trusted by the mostly Hispanic and immigrant population. The project maintained health equity at its center, and all decisions incorporated a human-centered design involving local residents, researchers, and public health experts to ensure applicability and relevance. Frequent meetings with TCP core members built trust and enabled us to pivot rapidly in the face of change.

EVALUATION AND ADVERSE EFFECTS

TCP used data triangulation, which involved collecting and analyzing quantitative and qualitative data and transforming data insights into action through the human-centered design. A clear indicator of success is the overall vaccine rate, which exceeded that of similar cities in Massachusetts; by mid-August 2021, the overall vaccination rate among adults exceeded 90% and ranked as one of the highest rates in the country for a city with similar demographics (Figure 1).[6]

Wastewater monitoring serves to detect changes in COVID-19 rates. These changes activated an on-the-ground response that included informing the public and distributing personal protective equipment and test kits. Given data indicating that the Omicron variant was surging in parts of Europe and evidence of increasing levels of COVID-19 specific to that variant, the Chelsea Board of Health passed a mask mandate in November 2021 by recommendation of TCP.

We are unaware of any adverse effects of this intervention.

SUSTAINABILITY

The collaboration activated by TCP provides a model for designing public health interventions. The diverse participants included data scientists and researchers, policymakers and state employees, CBOs, and local outreach workers. The diversity of the composition of TCP participants enables a 360-degree view of the problem, produces a variety of solutions, and improves equity in program design.

PUBLIC HEALTH SIGNIFICANCE

We lack surveillance data to estimate the true community case counts because some free, publicly available polymerase chain reaction test sites closed and at-home testing goes unreported. Wastewater testing allows passive surveillance, which provides early data on changes in levels of COVID-19

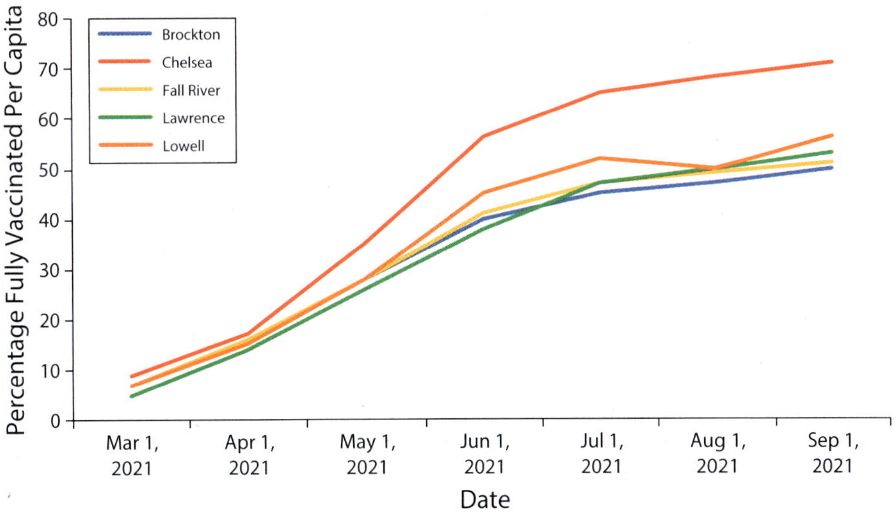

FIGURE 1— Full Vaccination Rates (Both Initial Doses) in Chelsea, MA, and Nearby Cities With Similar Demographics: 2021

Source: Massachusetts Department of Public Health.[6]

transmission and can enable public health–aligned community and municipal decision making in an evidence-informed manner.[7] Expanding wastewater testing to other infectious diseases is a promising new area.[8]

Human-centered design by communities enables projects to create solutions that are relevant, meaningful, and applicable. Through local CBOs, TCP consulted with the community on how to make information, education, and access trustworthy and streamlined.

The continuum of research into action through diverse stakeholders could inform the design and implementation of other projects. TCP was unique in Massachusetts in sharing results of data collected among those most affected by a disease, in turn empowering them to make decisions regarding their health in trusted spaces. In a time of increased urgency to design equitable responses,[9] TCP provides a blueprint for improving the lives of the most vulnerable. AJPH

ABOUT THE AUTHORS

Cristina Alonso is with the Harvard T. H. Chan School of Public Health, Boston, MA; La Colaborativa, Chelsea, MA; and the Center of Complex Interventions, Wellesley, MA. Barry Keppard is with the Metropolitan Area Planning Council, Boston. Samantha Bates is with the Center of Complex Interventions, Boston. Dan Cortez is with the Chelsea Police Department, Chelsea. Flor Amaya is with the Chelsea Department of Public Health, Chelsea. Karthik Dinakar is with Brigham and Women's Hospital, Boston; Massachusetts General Hospital, Boston; and the Massachusetts Institute of Technology Media Lab, Cambridge.

CORRESPONDENCE

Correspondence should be sent to Cristina Alonso, DrPH, MPH, CPM, 122 Bowdoin St, Apartment 107, Boston, MA 02108 (e-mail: cris@centerofci.org). Reprints can be ordered at http://www.ajph.org by clicking the "Reprints" link.

PUBLICATION INFORMATION

Full Citation: Alonso C, Keppard B, Bates S, Cortez D, Amaya F, Dinakar K. The Chelsea project: turning research and wastewater surveillance on COVID-19 into health equity action, Massachusetts, 2020–2021. *Am J Public Health*. 2023;113(6):627–630.

Acceptance Date: February 4, 2023.

DOI: https://doi.org/10.2105/AJPH.2023.307253

CONTRIBUTORS

C. Alonso and S. Bates conceptualized the article. C. Alonso wrote and revised the article. S. Bates and B. Keppard contributed to revising the article. B. Keppard designed the data visualization. S. Bates, D. Cortez, and K. Dinakar conceptualized the project. All of the authors participated in project implementation.

ACKNOWLEDGMENTS

We thank the Reid Hoffman Foundation for its support. Also, we thank La Colaborativa, Greenroots, Chelsea Black Community, Chelsea City Hall, and the Chelsea residents for their hard work during the pandemic.

CONFLICTS OF INTEREST

The authors have no conflicts of interest to declare.

HUMAN PARTICIPANT PROTECTION

The actions described in this article are not subject to protocol approval because no research involving human participants was conducted.

REFERENCES

1. Alonso C. The impact and social response to COVID-19 in Chelsea, Massachusetts. Available at: https://dash.harvard.edu/handle/1/37367919. Accessed June 17, 2020.
2. *Boston Globe* Editorial Board. Low-balling the Chelsea population threatens the state's coronavirus epicenter. Available at: https://www.bostonglobe.com/2020/06/14/opinion/an-undercounted-population-threatens-chelsea-states-coronavirus-epicenter. Accessed June 17, 2020.
3. Saltzman J. Nearly a third of 200 blood samples taken in Chelsea show exposure to coronavirus. Available at: https://www.bostonglobe.com/2020/04/17/business/nearly-third-200-blood-samples-taken-chelsea-show-exposure-coronavirus. Accessed January 29, 2021.
4. Barry E. In a crowded city, leaders struggle to separate the sick from the well. Available at: https://www.nytimes.com/2020/04/25/us/coronavirus-chelsea-massachusetts.html. Accessed July 6, 2020.
5. Massachusetts Department of Public Health. Weekly COVID-19 public health report: June 10, 2020. Available at: https://www.mass.gov/doc/weekly-covid-19-public-health-report-june-10-2020/download. Accessed June 12, 2020.
6. Massachusetts Department of Public Health. Archive of COVID-19 vaccination reports. Available at: https://www.mass.gov/info-details/archive-of-covid-19-vaccination-reports-2020-2021. Accessed January 23, 2023.
7. Aguiar-Oliveira ML, Campos AR, Matos A, et al. Wastewater-based epidemiology (WBE) and viral detection in polluted surface water: a valuable tool for COVID-19 surveillance—a brief review. *Int J Environ Res Public Health*. 2020;17(24):9251. https://doi.org/10.3390/ijerph17249251
8. Jiménez-Rodríguez MG, Silva-Lance F, Parra-Arroyo L, et al. Biosensors for the detection of disease outbreaks through wastewater-based epidemiology. *Trends Analyt Chem*. 2022;155:116585. https://doi.org/10.1016/j.trac.2022.116585
9. Berger ZD, Evans NG, Phelan AL, Silverman RD. Covid-19: control measures must be equitable and inclusive. *BMJ*. 2020;368:m1141. https://doi.org/10.1136/bmj.m1141

The Other Side of the Balance Sheet: Work as a Fundamental Determinant of Health

Devan Hawkins, ScD

ABOUT THE AUTHOR

Devan Hawkins is with the Public Health Program, School of Arts and Sciences, Massachusetts College of Pharmacy and Health Sciences University, Boston, MA.

See also Leigh, p. 634 and Gaffney et al., p. 647.

As the first wave of the COVID-19 pandemic was reaching its crest in March 2020, an article in the *Boston Globe* described cases of COVID-19 among hospital workers:

> Major hospitals in Boston are seeing a steep rise in the number of infected workers, a doubling to more than 160 in the past two days, which officials believe may be more attributable to community spread than contact with infected patients.[1]

This attribution of most cases among health care workers to community spread was echoed in quotations from hospital representatives, who argued that these cases were not predominately owing to occupational exposure. It was only in the second half of the article that the perspective of many health care workers was offered, when David Schildmeier from the Massachusetts Nurses Association was quoted as saying: "It's not safe for the nurses. They know they are putting themselves at risk, but they have no other choice."[1]

Such debates about the role of workplace transmission of COVID-19 have continued since the early days of the pandemic and expanded to include industries and occupations outside health care. Even as numerous studies have documented elevated rates of cases[2] and mortality[3,4] among high-exposure workers, a familiar refrain has been heard: how do we know that the infections were acquired at work? Because many of these studies used data that did not allow controlling for a wide-range of covariates that may be associated with COVID-19 infection, adequately answering this question was not always possible.

WORK-RELATED INFECTIONS

Fortunately, the new study from Gaffney et al. in this issue of *AJPH* (p. 647) provides strong evidence for the fundamental role that workplace transmission played in differences in the risk of COVID-19 infection. Using data from the nationally representative National Health Interview Survey, Gaffney et al. show that disparities in COVID-19 infection persist between certain industries and occupations even when controlling for covariates that may be associated with COVID-19 infection: age, gender, household size, and family income. In particular, the authors found that when this adjustment is performed, compared with workers in other industries and occupations, workers in the health care and social assistance industry and in health care practitioners and technical, health care support, and protective services occupations had significantly elevated rates of COVID-19. Workers in even more industries and occupations had significantly elevated rates of COVID-19 when nonworking adults were treated as the reference group.

The authors also show that the impact of occupational transmission of COVID-19 likely extends beyond the workers themselves. In their study, COVID-19 was positively correlated with the number of working people in the household. In an adjusted analysis, compared with households with no workers, households with one worker had a 26% higher risk of COVID-19, households with two workers had a 41% higher risk, and households with three or more workers had a 70% higher risk. This impact of workplace exposures on the health of household members has been seen with respect to other occupational exposures.[5] Another such example can be seen with parental leave. The United States is one of the only countries globally that does not mandate some form of paid parental leave. Studies have shown that there are health benefits of such policies for both the working parent and the child.[6]

DENYING THE ROLE OF WORK

The article by Gaffney et al. is an important contribution to the wide literature about the role that work plays in the risk of disease, injury, and death. This role will often be denied by management and ownership. For example, for years the asbestos industry covered up the links between its products and lung diseases, including cancers.[7]

The reasons for such denial are clear. Under the Occupational Health and Safety Act of 1970's General Duty Clause, each employer is required to "furnish to each of his employees employment and a place of employment which are free from recognized hazards that are causing or are likely to cause death or serious physical harm to his employees."[8] If you can show that an illness like COVID-19, other diseases, or injuries are caused by work then the employer has an obligation to prevent those exposures and protect workers. In a profit-driven economy, efforts to protect workers' health and safety will often be seen as a cost sink. At a time when some businesses are so desperate for cheap employment that child labor law violations have increased by 69% since 2018,[9] it should not come as a surprise that the health and safety of workers will be disregarded.

We saw similar disregard for the well-being of workers during last year's railroad labor dispute, when railroad industry workers tried to negotiate more paid sick leave days. Lack of paid sick leave is a problem across industries and occupations in the United States, and indeed many of the occupations identified as having elevated risk for COVID-19 in the study by Gaffney et al. have lower access to paid sick leave than other workers.[10] Although the assumption that offering paid sick leave is bad for profits may be false, as a recent literature review found,[11] the prospect of laws mandating access to this important benefit still seem unlikely.

INVESTING IN WORKER PROTECTION

Gaffney et al. have provided more evidence for the role of work as a fundamental determinant of health. The fact that work is such a fundamental determinant of health should not be a surprise. Adults spend much of their waking hours at work. Studies like that of Gaffney et al., which isolate the role of work, are particularly important. Understanding that work contributes to disparities in a wide variety of health outcomes gives a clear target for interventions to prevent those health outcomes. Fortunately, there are means by which work as a fundamental determinant of health can be targeted. As Gaffney et al. refer to in their article, the Occupational Safety and Health Administration (OSHA) is an entire agency tasked with protecting workers and ensuring safe workplaces. However, as the authors also describe, despite growth in complaints to OSHA in 2020, inspections fell. Difficulty in carrying out inspections has been a persistent problem for OSHA. One analysis suggested that with the number of inspectors employed by the agency, it would take 129 years to inspect each workplace in the country.[12]

Protecting workers from infectious diseases, injuries, chemical hazards, and psychosocial exposures at work requires an investment in agencies like OSHA so that they can fulfill their mission as well as an understanding of why the health and well-being of workers is so often disregarded. Whether it is a health care facility administrator skimping on adequate personal protective equipment (e.g., face masks, goggles, gloves) for workers, a warehouse manager refusing to give an employee a paid day off so they can get therapy for chronic pain from occupational lifting, or a boss saying that there is not enough time for that one last safety check, attempts to protect health and prevent death and injury are seen as a threat to the bottom line. Profit. Health is on the other side of the balance sheet. AJPH

CORRESPONDENCE

Correspondence should be sent to Devan Hawkins, 179 Longwood Ave, Boston, MA 02115 (e-mail: devan.hawkins@mcphs.edu). Reprints can be ordered at http://www.ajph.org by clicking the "Reprints" link.

PUBLICATION INFORMATION

Full Citation: Hawkins D. The other side of the balance sheet: work as a fundamental determinant of health. *Am J Public Health*. 2023;113(6): 631–633.

Acceptance Date: March 20, 2023.

DOI: https://doi.org/10.2105/AJPH.2023.307300

ACKNOWLEDGMENTS

I would like to thank *AJPH* editor-in-chief, Alfredo Morabia, for the helpful feedback received for earlier drafts of this editorial.

CONFLICTS OF INTEREST

The author has no conflicts of interest to declare.

REFERENCES

1. Priyanka DM. More than 160 Boston hospital workers test positive for coronavirus: many appear to be due to community spread, as opposed to contact with infected patients. *Boston Globe*. March 26, 2020. Available at: https://www.bostonglobe.com/2020/03/26/metro/dozens-boston-hospital-staffers-have-contracted-coronavirus. Accessed March 22, 2023.
2. Heinzerling A, Nguyen A, Frederick M, et al. Workplaces most affected by COVID-19 outbreaks in California, January 2020–August 2021. *Am J Public Health*. 2022;112(8):1180–1190. https://doi.org/10.2105/AJPH.2022.306862
3. Billock RM, Steege AL, Miniño A. COVID-19 mortality by usual occupation and industry: 46 states and New York City, United States, 2020. *Natl Vital Stat Rep*. 2022;71(6):1–33. https://dx.doi.org/10.15620/cdc:120292
4. Hawkins D, Davis L, Kriebel D. COVID-19 deaths by occupation, Massachusetts, March 1–July 31, 2020. *Am J Ind Med*. 2021;64(4):238–244. https://doi.org/10.1002/ajim.23227
5. Kalweit A, Herrick RF, Flynn MA, et al. Eliminating take-home exposures: recognizing the role of occupational health and safety in broader community health. *Ann Work Expo Health*. 2020;64(3):236–249. https://doi.org/10.1093/annweh/wxaa006

6. Van Niel MS, Bhatia R, Riano NS, et al. The impact of paid maternity leave on the mental and physical health of mothers and children: a review of the literature and policy implications. *Harv Rev Psychiatry.* 2020;28(2):113–126. https://doi.org/10.1097/HRP.0000000000000246
7. Egilman D, Bird T, Lee C. Dust diseases and the legacy of corporate manipulation of science and law. *Int J Occup Environ Health.* 2014;20(2):115–125. https://doi.org/10.1179/1077352514Z.000000000104
8. Occupational Safety and Health Administration. OSH Act of 1970. Available at: https://www.osha.gov/laws-regs/oshact/section5-duties. Accessed March 14, 2023.
9. US Department of Labor. Departments of Labor, Health and Human Services announce new efforts to combat exploitative child labor. February 27, 2023. Available at: https://www.dol.gov/newsroom/releases/osec/osec20230227. Accessed March 14, 2023.
10. Hawkins D. Disparities in access to paid sick leave during the first year of the COVID-19 pandemic. *J Occup Environ Med.* 2023; Epub ahead of print. https://doi.org/10.1097/JOM.0000000000002784
11. Vander Weerdt C, Stoddard-Dare P, DeRigne L. Is paid sick leave bad for business? A systematic review. *Am J Ind Med.* 2023; Epub ahead of print. https://doi.org/10.1002/ajim.23469
12. American Federation of Labor and Congress of Industrial Organizations. Death on the job: the toll of neglect, 2011. April 28, 2011. Available at: https://aflcio.org/reports/death-job-2011. Accessed June 11, 2022.

COVID-19 May Have Been Job Related for One Fourth of Diagnosed Adults

J. Paul Leigh, PhD

ABOUT THE AUTHOR

The author is with the Department of Public Health Sciences and the Center for Healthcare Policy and Research, University of California, Davis, Medical School, and the Center for Poverty and Inequality Research, University of California, Davis.

See also Hawkins, p. 631 and Gaffney et al., p. 647.

AJPH June 2023, Vol 113, No. 6

We catch COVID-19 from each other. The fewer people we encounter, the safer we will be. Our desire for fewer encounters was especially apparent in employment arrangements during the first two and a half years of the pandemic. Most workers whom employers allowed to work from home did so; most whose employers did not allow this reported to their workplaces.

We labeled essential workers and recognized them as physicians, nurses, and police officers but also nursing home aides, warehouse workers, and meatpackers. In the first few months, we literally applauded health care workers and praised grocery store employers who offered hazardous pay to employees. As the months wore on, we became less mindful of essential workers; the applause and hazardous pay ended, but the virus did not. The virus revealed a chasm in the labor force between largely lower-paid (with the exception of health care professionals) essential workers and higher-paid nonessential workers. There was never any significant "shared sacrifice." This chasm, in fact, has always existed for occupational diseases; COVID-19 merely shined klieg lights on it.

COVID-19 INFECTIONS

Gaffney et al. (p. 647) provide the best estimate of this chasm to date. The Gaffney et al. study has advantages. Previous US studies relied on data from either Massachusetts or California. Gaffney and colleagues are the first to use the nationally representative National Health Interview Survey. Their sample size is large (46 321). A second advantage is that they use US government codes to classify occupations and industries, thereby allowing useful comparisons with occupational health, economic, and sociological studies that relied on these classifications.

In fact, their study can be viewed as an extension of a long line of research ranking occupations and industries according to measures including job-related injury fatalities[1] and mental illness.[2] Consistent with the Gaffney et al. findings, these job-ranking health studies revealed disproportionate burdens falling on African Americans, Hispanics, and low-wage workers.[1] Finally, no previous national study has compared people who have jobs with those who do not; the Gaffney et al. data can be used to calculate the population attributable fraction (PAF) in relation to contracting COVID-19 as a result of job-related exposures (as described subsequently).

Gaffney et al. confirm and expand on the findings of previous studies. The most dangerous jobs are in health care and public safety. Gaffney and colleagues' broad category of "health practitioners" includes physicians, registered nurses, and emergency medical technicians. The broad "health care support" category includes aides, orderlies, and home health care workers. The broad category of "protective service" includes police officers, firefighters, and prison guards, and the "community and social services" and "food preparation and serving" categories include social workers, probation officers, community organizers, food servers, kitchen staff, and meatpackers. To some extent, their findings mirror those of studies on workplace violence, which obviously apply to police personnel, guards, and probation officers. But less well known is that important causes of injuries to nurses, aides, social workers, and even physicians are unruly and violent patients and clients.[3] Meatpackers experience very high injury rates involving violence to animals.[4]

Low-risk occupations and industries include Gaffney and colleagues' broad "legal," "management," and "business and financial" categories. These categories involve those engaged in specific occupational roles, such as lawyers, managers, and bankers, all of whom could do much of their work from home.

These white-collar jobs also have low occupational injury and (non-COVID-19) illness rates.[1,4] In addition, although Gaffney et al. and other authors include farming and military jobs as relatively safe from COVID-19, these jobs have high injury and (non-COVID-19) illness rates.[1,4] It could be that work outdoors explains the low COVID-19 rates for farming and military jobs. Interestingly, in the Gaffney et al. study farming had the lowest percentage of workers reporting testing for COVID-19 (37.2%), whereas the military had the highest percentage (72.5%).

One limitation of the Gaffney et al. study is that the data pertain to infections rather than deaths. Most studies with data on deaths have shown that health care workers are not at the top of the list. Billock et al.[5] found the death rate for health care practitioners and technical workers to be significantly below the average for all occupations. A second limitation is that the Gaffney et al. categories are quite broad. Other studies have generated rankings of more informative specific jobs (e.g., janitors, clerks) with smaller overall sample sizes than are available in the National Health Interview Survey.[1,2]

POPULATION ATTRIBUTABLE FRACTIONS

Epidemiologists use PAFs to estimate disease burdens attributable to different factors. For example, 8% of cancer and 10% of chronic obstructive pulmonary disease cases are attributed to occupational exposures to carcinogens, dusts, and other toxins.[6] Gaffney et al. report that their sample included 28 267 "workers" and 18 054 "nonworkers" 18 years or older, of whom 12.4% and 8.1%, respectively, reported COVID-19 infections (personal communication, March 13, 2023); overall, 4977 people reported infections. Applying the PAF method, if workers had not had workplace exposures, the number of infected people would have been 3752 (8.1% × [18 054 + 28 267]). The "excess" number of infected people is 1225 (4977 − 3752). The PAF for COVID-19 is 24.6% (1225/4977). This PAF is higher than any other occupational PAFs other than that for pneumoconiosis (black lung, asbestosis, and silicosis).[6] I believe that this is the first national job-related PAF estimate for COVID-19.

SIGNIFICANCE

As time goes on, as more people go back to their workplaces, and as the virus spreads to infect the entire population, the chasm across occupations and the PAF for the occupational contribution will shrink somewhat; however, both will likely remain significant as with other occupational diseases. The Gaffney et al. study is a fresh reminder that work, where most adults spend 40% or more of their waking hours, is a critical social determinant of health and involves health equity issues.[5,7]

COVID-19 in the workplace has other implications. Legal debates are under way pertaining to workers' compensation. If other occupational diseases are any guide, workers' compensation insurers will find ways to avoid paying 80% to 99% of the costs, thereby passing the financial burden along to other private health insurers, Medicaid and Medicare (i.e., taxpayers), and the afflicted families.[6] COVID-19 is likely partially responsible for the surge in public interest in labor unions and increasing strike activity since 2019.[8] Christian Smalls, the leader of the new Amazon Labor Union in New York, attributes his activism to management's disregard for the well-being of warehouse workers. Occupational hazards are well-known predictors of union formation and strikes.[9]

Finally, Gaffney et al. report no funding for their study; this is typical for occupational health research. Even though the economic burden of occupational injuries and illnesses is on par with cancer,[10] one of the lowest levels of funding in the National Institutes of Health is that for the National Institute for Occupational Safety and Health (NIOSH). (Technically, NIOSH is part of the Centers for Disease Control and Prevention.) Twenty institutes have more funding, and typically much more. For instance, the fiscal year 2023 National Cancer Institute budget is $6.714 billion, 17 times larger than the NIOSH $396 million budget; the National Institute on Aging budget ($4.011 billion) is 10 times larger, and the budget for the Office of the Director ($2.413 billion) is six times larger. The NIOSH budget is less than that of the National Library of Medicine ($472 million).[11] AJPH

CORRESPONDENCE

Correspondence should be sent to J. Paul Leigh, PhD, Department of Public Health Sciences, UC Davis, Davis, CA 95616 (e-mail: pleigh@ucdavis.edu). Reprints can be ordered at http://www.ajph.org by clicking the "Reprints" link.

PUBLICATION INFORMATION

Full Citation: Leigh JP. COVID-19 may have been job related for one fourth of diagnosed adults. *Am J Public Health*. 2023;113(6):634–636.

Acceptance Date: March 20, 2023.

DOI: https://doi.org/10.2105/AJPH.2023.307299

ACKNOWLEDGMENTS

I thank Regina Pana-Cryan for providing information on National Institutes of Health budgets.

CONFLICTS OF INTEREST

The author received funding from the National Institute for Occupational Safety and Health from 2008 to 2011.

REFERENCES

1. US Department of Labor, Bureau of Labor Statistics. Census of fatal occupational injuries in 2021. Available at: https://www.bls.gov/news.release/pdf/cfoi.pdf. Accessed March 13, 2023.
2. Eaton WW, Anthony JC, Mandel W, Garrison R. Occupations and the prevalence of major depressive disorder. *J Occup Med.* 1990;32(11):1079–1087. https://doi.org/10.1097/00043764-199011000-00006
3. Piquero NL, Piquero AR, Craig JM, Clipper SJ. Assessing research on workplace violence, 2000–2012. *Aggress Violent Behav.* 2013;18(3):383–394. https://doi.org/10.1016/j.avb.2013.03.001
4. US Department of Labor, Bureau of Labor Statistics. Injuries and illnesses. Available at: https://www.bls.gov/iif. Accessed March 14, 2023.
5. Billock R, Steege A, Miniño A. COVID-19 Mortality by usual occupation and industry: 46 states and New York City, United States, 2020. Available at: https://stacks.cdc.gov/view/cdc/120292. Accessed March 14, 2023.
6. Leigh JP, Robbins JA. Occupational disease and workers' compensation: coverage, costs, and consequences. *Milbank Q.* 2004;82(4):689–721. https://doi.org/10.1111/j.0887-378X.2004.00328.x
7. Wolfe R, Hartnett K, Schneider D. Inequalities at work and the toll of COVID-19. Available at: https://www.healthaffairs.org/do/10.1377/hpb20210428.863621/full. Accessed March 14, 2023.
8. McCarthy J. US approval of labor unions at highest point since 1965. Available at: https://news.gallup.com/poll/398303/approval-labor-unions-highest-point-1965.aspx. Accessed March 13, 2023.
9. Pouliakas K, Theodossiou I. The economics of health and safety at work: an interdisciplinary review of the theory and policy. *J Econ Surv.* 2013;27(1):167–208. https://doi.org/10.1111/j.1467-6419.2011.00699.x
10. Leigh JP. Economic burden of occupational injury and illness in the United States. *Milbank Q.* 2011;89(4):728–772. https://doi.org/10.1111/j.1468-0009.2011.00648.x
11. US Department of Health and Human Services. Fiscal year 2023 budget in brief. Available at: https://www.hhs.gov/sites/default/files/fy-2023-budget-in-brief.pdf. Accessed March 13, 2023.

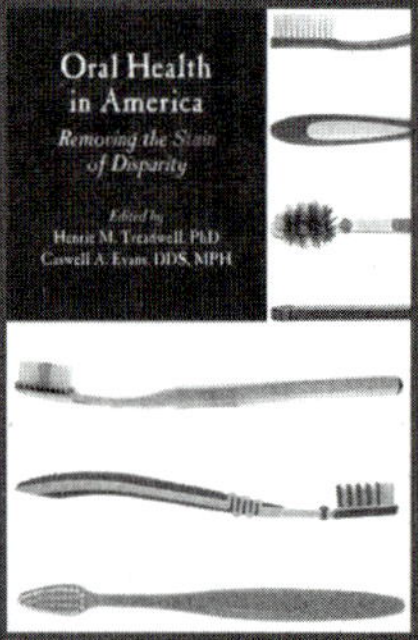

Dead Labor: Mortality Inequities by Class, Gender, and Race/Ethnicity in the United States, 1986–2019

Jerzy Eisenberg-Guyot, PhD, MPH, Megan C. Finsaas, PhD, MA, and Seth J. Prins, PhD, MPH

Objectives. To estimate social class inequities in US mortality using a relational measure based on power over productive property and workers' labor.

Methods. We used nationally representative 1986–2018 National Health Interview Survey data with mortality follow-up through December 31, 2019 (n = 911 850). First, using business-ownership, occupational, and employment-status data, we classified respondents as incorporated business owners (IBOs), unincorporated business owners (UBOs), managers, workers, or not in the labor force (NLFs). Next, using inverse-probability-weighted survival curves, we estimated class mortality inequities overall, after subdividing workers by employment status and occupation, and by period, gender, race/ethnicity, and education.

Results. UBOs, workers, and NLFs had, respectively, 6.3 (95% confidence interval [CI] = −8.1, −4.6), 6.6 (95% CI = −8.1, −5.0), and 19.4 (95% CI = −21.0, −17.7) per 100 lower 34-year survival rates than IBOs. Mortality risk was especially high for unemployed, blue-collar, and service workers. Inequities increased over time and were greater among male, racially minoritized, and less-educated respondents.

Conclusions. We estimated considerable mortality inequities by class, gender, and race/ethnicity. We also estimated that class mortality inequities are increasing, threatening population health.

Public Health Implications. Addressing class inequities likely requires structural, worker-empowering interventions. (*Am J Public Health*. 2023;113(6):637–646. https://doi.org/10.2105/AJPH.2023.307227)

AJPH June 2023, Vol 113, No. 6

"Capital is dead labour, which, vampire-like, lives only by sucking living labour, and lives the more, the more labour it sucks."

—*Karl Marx*[1(p342)]

Mining the abyss of 19th century capitalism, Marx unearthed capitalism's deadly structural logic: the material welfare and security of the owning class depends on the deprivation and alienation of the working class and dispossessed.[1(pp340–416),2] Much subsequent epidemiological research has documented health inequities across social positions defined by socioeconomic indicators like income, education, occupation, and working conditions.[2] However, by treating social positions as individual-level attributes rather than as constituted by social relations, the research has elided the structural relationships, such as differences in economic power, that produce social positions and ultimately cause health inequities.[2,3] Here, we return to Marx. Leveraging 1986–2018 National Health Interview Survey (NHIS) data, we apply a relational social class theory based on power over productive property and workers' labor to analyze US mortality inequities by class, gender, and race/ethnicity. Only a relational theory, which recognizes that the material welfare of some groups causally depends on the deprivation of others,[4] can identify the root causes of health inequities across social positions. Such root causes may be more efficient and effective targets for public health intervention than downstream, individual-level factors.[5]

RELATIONAL SOCIAL CLASS AND HEALTH INEQUITIES

Tapping Marxist theories, we define social class in terms of power over labor and productive property (i.e., the tangible and intangible assets used to make commodities).[2–4,6] Capitalists (e.g., business owners), who constitute a minority of the population, own productive property, control workers' labor processes (dominating them), and appropriate as surplus the difference in value between what workers produce and what they are compensated (exploiting them).[2,3,6] Conversely, workers, who constitute a majority of the population, lack productive property and survive by selling their labor power to capitalists for a wage.[2,3,6] The inversely interdependent relationship between capitalists and workers is the root cause of many socioeconomic health inequities.[2,3,5] Indeed, capitalists' productive property is derived from the undercompensated output of workers' past, dead labor, and their profits and accumulating wealth flow from the ongoing exploitation and domination of workers' current, living labor.[1(pp340–416)] Thus, the material well-being of capitalists requires workers' deprivation, subjugation, and overexertion,[2,3,5] which is wrought by the drive to increase surplus extraction, absolutely (e.g., prolonging working hours) or relatively (e.g., debasing wages and working conditions).[1(p432)]

Additional class relationships beyond capitalists and workers also affect health and well-being.[3–5,7] For example, the petite bourgeoisie (e.g., independent shopkeepers) own some productive property but labor themselves rather than controlling workers' labor.[3–5,7] Although the petite bourgeoisie often have considerable control over their working lives, they may lack sufficient resources to compete with capitalists, elevating their risk of business failure, stress, and poverty.[8] Conversely, most managers lack productive property, but they supervise workers' labor at capitalists' behest, exercising delegated ownership authority.[3–5,7] Although high-level managers or executives may resemble capitalists by enjoying considerable compensation, ownership stakes (e.g., stocks), autonomy, and authority (i.e., less domination and exploitation), low-level managers may be simultaneously exploited and dominated by management and face antagonism from subordinates, inducing stress and other hazards.[7] Consequently, the petite bourgeoisie's and low-level managers' health risks may resemble or exceed workers', a phenomenon difficult to identify or explain with gradational, stratificationist theories of social position that predict linear class-outcome relationships (e.g., the "socioeconomic gradient").[3,7,8]

Class relations interact with structural sexism and racism to produce health inequities.[9–13] Women and racialized people, especially those who are Black, Indigenous, Hispanic, or undocumented, are segregated into the working class.[5] There, they are further segregated into hyperexploited employment, including service work and hazardous blue-collar occupations, where they face high rates of workplace sexism, racism, and other forms of discrimination.[9–13] This discrimination has health-harming material and psychosocial consequences such as poverty and chronic stress.[9–13] Minoritized people are also disproportionately segregated into unemployment,[10] where they cycle into and out of precarious, low-wage jobs,[14] or they are excluded from waged labor entirely because of disability (often precipitated by work-related injuries),[13] incarceration,[10] or unpaid domestic labor.[15]

Changes in the balance of power across classes also shape health inequities.[5] Since the 1980s, power in the United States has tipped further away from workers. From 1989 to 2020, union density dropped from 16% to 11%, including from 22% to 12% among non-Hispanic Black workers.[16] Plummeting union density has eroded workers' power over wages and working conditions.[17,18] Indeed, the ratio of mean income among the top 1% versus the bottom 50% of earners grew from 27 to 81 from 1980 to 2015.[19] Surging mortality disparities across socioeconomic groups defined by income, education, and other factors[20] may reflect employers' consolidating class power.

RESEARCH GAPS AND OBJECTIVES

A small but growing body of US research has identified social class relations as drivers of numerous health outcomes, including self-rated health, mental illness, and substance use.[2,3] Yet, despite well-theorized and empirically supported mechanisms linking class relations to mortality inequities, few US-based studies have applied relational theories to investigate the topic. Moreover, to our knowledge, no studies have examined temporal changes in class mortality inequities, a substantial gap given burgeoning mortality disparities across other social axes.

Data limitations have impeded previous research, as epidemiological data sets rarely contain detailed social class and mortality data, let alone adequate sample sizes to precisely estimate inequities within time periods, genders, or races/ethnicities.[18] A few previous

US-based studies estimated considerable class mortality inequities, but they were conducted decades ago or had imprecise findings.[21,22]

We addressed these gaps by applying a relational social class theory to nationally representative 1986–2018 NHIS data linked to the National Death Index (NDI) through 2019. Our specific objectives were to (1) estimate the magnitude of class mortality inequities among working-age adults from 1986 to 2018, (2) analyze changes in such inequities over time, and (3) identify how class mortality inequities vary within and across genders, races/ethnicities, and socioeconomic subgroups.

METHODS

The NHIS is a repeated cross-sectional, nationally representative survey of the noninstitutionalized US population conducted by the US Census Bureau on behalf of the National Center for Health Statistics.[23] The NHIS has collected sociodemographic and health data since 1957.[23] From 1997 to 2018, household response rates were 64% to 92%.[23] Respondents aged 18 years and older in the 1986–2018 survey are linked to the NDI using available identifying information (e.g., social security number, names, birth date, gender, race, birth location, and state of residence), with mortality follow-up through December 31, 2019.[24] For select records, synthetic data are substituted for date of death to reduce disclosure risk; mortality status is unperturbed.[24]

For our analyses, we used harmonized 1986–2018 NHIS data from the Integrated Public Use Microdata Series.[25] We then made sample restrictions. First, we excluded respondents younger than 25 or older than 64 years to focus on populations with high labor-force attachment.[22] Next, we addressed data issues. First, we excluded the 1997–2000 survey waves and non–sample adults from 2001 to 2018, as such waves and respondents lacked complete social class data. Second, we excluded respondents with insufficient identifying information for NDI linkage (< 3%). Third, per the advice of NHIS administrators, we excluded the 1992 Hispanic oversample (< 0.5%).[24] Finally, we excluded respondents (< 3%) with missing exposure or covariate data. Appendix A1 (available as a supplement to the online version of this article at http://www.ajph.org) contains a flow diagram.

Our analyses used NHIS eligibility-adjusted sampling weights to make estimates nationally representative and address linkage ineligibility, nonresponse, and oversampling.[24] We conducted our analyses in R version 4.1.0 (R Foundation for Statistical Computing, Vienna, Austria). Our code is available on GitHub (https://github.com/Critical-Social-Epi/NHIS_class_mortality).

Measures

Social class. To measure social class, we used data on respondents' employment status, as well as their business-ownership status and occupation as proxies for power over productive property and labor.[8,26] First, those not in the labor force (NLFs) were those who identified their employment status in the past 1 to 2 weeks as "not in the labor force." Second, workers were those who identified as unemployed or as an employee with a nonexecutive, nonadministrative, and nonmanagerial occupation. We classified the unemployed as workers because many precarious workers cycle between employment and unemployment.[8,14] Although NLFs may also cycle into and out of employment, especially into working-class employment, others may remain out of the labor force because of disability, retirement, domestic-labor responsibilities, or otherwise.[8,14] Third, managers were those who identified as an employee with an executive, administrative, or managerial occupation. Finally, unincorporated business owners (UBOs) were those who identified as self-employed in an unincorporated business, whereas incorporated business owners (IBOs) were those who identified as self-employed in an incorporated business. An incorporated business (i.e., corporation) is a shareholder-owned independent legal entity that is itself liable for business actions and debts,[27] unlike unincorporated businesses, whose proprietors remain liable. Although incorporation provides legal protections and tax benefits, smaller businesses use it less frequently than larger ones because of administrative costs and complexities.[27,28] Indeed, in 2015, 41% of IBOs employed workers versus just 13% of UBOs[27]; moreover, IBOs have higher mean incomes.[28] This suggests that IBOs are more likely to be capitalists than UBOs, although many IBOs do not employ workers and thus are not capitalists. Therefore, we refrain from referring to IBOs and UBOs as "capitalists" and "petite bourgeoisie," despite overlap. Appendix A2 (available as a supplement to the online version of this article at http://www.ajph.org) contains questionnaire wording and a decision tree.

Mortality. Mortality status and death year (if applicable) were available for all respondents eligible for NDI linkage.[24] For the deceased, we calculated follow-up time by subtracting the interview year from the death year, assuming the

AJPH June 2023, Vol 113, No. 6

interview happened at the beginning of each year and deaths occurred at the end of each year. For those living through December 31, 2019, we calculated follow-up time by subtracting the interview year from 2020. We calculated follow-up time at the year level for simplicity and to increase the stability of our estimates.

Covariates. Covariates of interest included respondents' age, race/ethnicity (self-identified), gender (generally assigned by the interviewer based on respondents' first names or relationship to household head), education, region of residence, and interview year.

Analyses

First, we estimated class-stratified descriptive statistics of our sample. We also characterized the class composition of each gender–race/ethnicity group and the gender–race/ethnicity composition of each class, and estimated the yearly proportion of respondents in each class.

Next, we estimated class mortality inequities using inverse-probability-weighted survival curves and Cox proportional hazards models.[29] First, we estimated the inverse probability weights (IPW). For a given respondent, the IPW numerator was the unconditional probability of belonging to their observed class in the sample, and the denominator was the conditional probability of belonging to their observed class, given their confounder values. Using R's "ipw" package,[30] we estimated the numerator and denominator probabilities using multinomial logistic regression models with social class outcomes, weighted by the NHIS's sampling weights.[31] The numerator model contained only the intercept as a predictor, and the denominator contained predictors of gender, age, and interview year (with the latter 2 specified as 3-knot and 5-knot restricted cubic splines, respectively). Next, we multiplied together the IPW and NHIS sampling weights.[31] Finally, using the combined weights and R's "survival" package,[32] we ran inverse-probability-weighted Kaplan–Meier survival curves with robust standard errors and a years-since-baseline timescale, which estimated the probability of survival over follow-up by class and the difference in the probability of survival (survival difference [SVD]) at the end of follow-up (34 years) in each class relative to the probability of survival among IBOs.[29] We estimated standard errors (SEs) for the SVDs as follows[33]:

$$SE_{SVD} = \sqrt{(SE_{Probability\ of\ survival\ in\ given\ class})^2 + (SE_{Probability\ of\ survival\ in\ IBOs})^2} \quad (1)$$

Using "survival,"[32] we also ran inverse-probability-weighted Cox models with robust standard errors and a years-since-baseline timescale, which estimated the mortality hazard across follow-up among each class relative to IBOs' hazard.[29] Because the survival curves and Cox models were inverse probability weighted, their estimates were nationally representative and adjusted for confounding by age, gender, and interview year.[29] In our primary analyses, we did not adjust for additional confounders via the IPW to capture the total magnitude of class inequities, including inequities reflecting the segregation of minoritized and oppressed respondents into more exploited and dominated classes.[5]

We also estimated the IPW, survival curves, and Cox models (1) after subdividing "workers" by employment status and occupation (i.e., unemployed workers, service workers, blue-collar workers [production, craft, and repair; operator, fabricator, and laborer; farming, forestry, and fishing; and military occupations], and white-collar workers [professional–specialty and technical, sales, and administrative-support occupations]); (2) within time periods (1986–1996 waves with follow-up through December 31, 2004, vs 2001–2018 waves with follow-up through December 31, 2019); and (3) after interacting class with gender (women vs men), race/ethnicity (non-Hispanic Black, Hispanic, and non-Hispanic "other" vs non-Hispanic White), and educational attainment (≤ high school vs > high school).

RESULTS

Our sample (n = 911 850) was 2% IBOs, 6% UBOs, 10% managers, 61% workers, and 21% NLFs (Table 1), a structure that was mostly stable from 1986 to 2018 (Appendix A3, available as a supplement to the online version of this article at http://www.ajph.org). Workers constituted over half of each gender–race/ethnicity group (online Appendix A3). Nonetheless, we identified gendered and racialized labor segregation, with non-Hispanic White men more likely to be IBOs, UBOs, or managers (25%) than other gender–races/ethnicities, especially than non-Hispanic Black women (10%; online Appendix A3). Consequently, workers and NLFs were disproportionately women and racially minoritized; they were also disproportionately unmarried and were less educated than IBOs and managers (Table 1). IBOs and managers, meanwhile, were disproportionately non-Hispanic White, more educated, and married; IBOs were also disproportionately men (Table 1). Fifty-two percent of workers had white-collar occupations, 14% had service occupations, 27% had blue-collar occupations, and 7% were unemployed (online Appendix A3).

Our sample included 170 834 deaths over 18 350 369 follow-up years.

TABLE 1— Sociodemographic Composition of Sample, Stratified by Social Class: National Health Interview Survey, United States, 1986–2018

	IBOs	UBOs	Managers	Workers	NLFs
Total, %	2.3	6.0	10.0	60.6	21.1
Women, %	27.5	39.0	45.9	47.7	69.7
Race/ethnicity, %					
Hispanic	6.8	10.9	7.3	13.2	13.6
Non-Hispanic Black	4.2	5.9	8.0	12.5	12.9
Non-Hispanic other	5.8	4.6	5.4	5.4	5.6
Non-Hispanic White	83.2	78.7	79.3	68.8	68.0
Education, %					
< high school	4.7	12.3	2.0	11.0	22.7
High school	23.3	33.2	17.1	32.5	34.8
Some college	26.3	26.4	25.3	27.8	24.1
College or more	45.7	28.2	55.6	28.7	18.4
Marital status, %					
Married	80.9	72.6	70.4	64.3	66.0
Single	8.3	12.4	15.3	19.2	14.9
Widowed/divorced/separated	10.9	15.0	14.2	16.5	19.1
Region, %					
Midwest	23.1	23.3	23.4	24.5	21.5
Northeast	19.3	16.5	19.9	18.9	18.2
South	36.3	34.0	34.4	35.4	38.1
West	21.3	26.3	22.3	21.2	22.2
Age, median (IQR[a])	46 (38, 54)	45 (36, 53)	42 (34, 51)	41 (32, 50)	49 (36, 59)
Interview year, median (IQR[a])	2005 (1994, 2012)	2003 (1992, 2010)	2006 (1995, 2013)	2006 (1994, 2012)	2006 (1994, 2012)

Note. IBOs = incorporated business owners; IQR = interquartile range; NLFs = those not in the labor force; UBOs = unincorporated business owners. Estimates are based on survey-weighted data from respondents aged 25–64 years to the United States' 1986–2018 National Health Interview Survey (n = 911 850).
[a]Interquartile range (quartile 1, quartile 3).

Respondents were followed for a median and maximum of 24 and 34 years, respectively. Appendix A4 (available as a supplement to the online version of this article at http://www.ajph.org) contains IPW distributions.

We estimated considerable class mortality inequities (Figure 1 and Appendix A5, available as a supplement to the online version of this article at http://www.ajph.org). Indeed, UBOs, workers, and NLFs had, respectively, 6.3 (95% confidence interval [CI] = −8.1, −4.6), 6.6 (95% CI = −8.1, −5.0), and 19.4 (95% CI = −21.0, −17.7) per 100 lower 34-year survival rates than IBOs. Managers fared similarly to IBOs. Blue-collar, service, and unemployed workers were at especially increased mortality risk, whereas white-collar workers fared similarly to IBOs and managers. Inequities lessened but persisted in further-adjusted analyses (gender, age, and year, plus education, marital status, region, and race/ethnicity; online Appendix A5). Including the Hispanic oversample did not meaningfully alter estimates, nor did alternative standard-error-estimation approaches (online Appendix A5).

We estimated that the class mortality inequities increased over time (Figure 2 and Appendix A6, available as a supplement to the online version of this article at http://www.ajph.org). For example, in the 1986–1996 waves with follow-up through December 31, 2004, only NLFs had a meaningfully lower 19-year survival rate than IBOs (SVD per 100 = −11.0; 95% CI = −12.7, −9.3). However, in the 2001–2018 waves with follow-up through December 31, 2019, UBOs, workers, and NLFs had, respectively, 3.5 (95% CI = −5.2, −1.7), 2.9 (95% CI = −4.3, −1.4), and 14.9 (95% CI = −16.6, −13.3) per 100 lower 19-year survival rates than IBOs. The estimated growth in mortality inequities persisted in more-adjusted analyses and appeared greater in Cox models incorporating class-by-interview-year

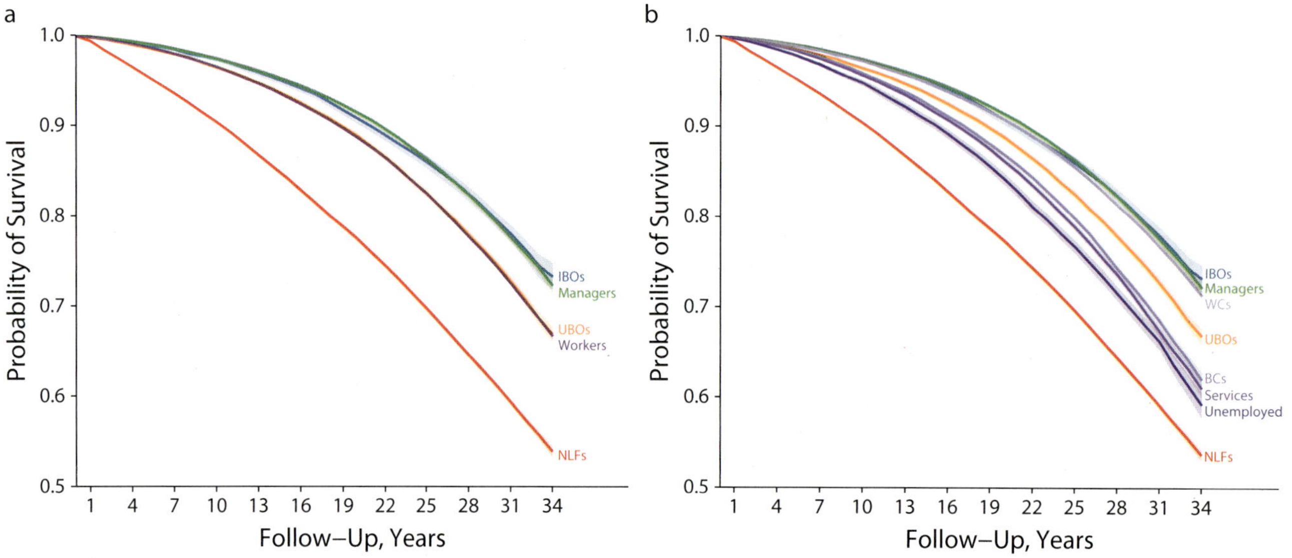

FIGURE 1— **Inverse-Probability-Weighted Kaplan–Meier Survival Curves Depicting Probability of Survival During Follow-Up (a) by Class Overall and (b) After Subdividing Workers by Occupation and Employment Status: United States**

Note. BCs = blue-collar workers; IBOs = incorporated business owners; NLFs = those not in the labor force; UBOs = unincorporated business owners; WCs = white-collar workers. Curves estimated on sample of respondents aged 25–64 years to the United States' 1986–2018 National Health Interview Survey (NHIS) with mortality follow-up through December 31, 2019 (n = 911 850). Via inverse probability weighting, estimates from curves are nationally representative and adjusted for gender, age, and interview year. Ninety-five percent confidence bands estimated with robust standard errors.

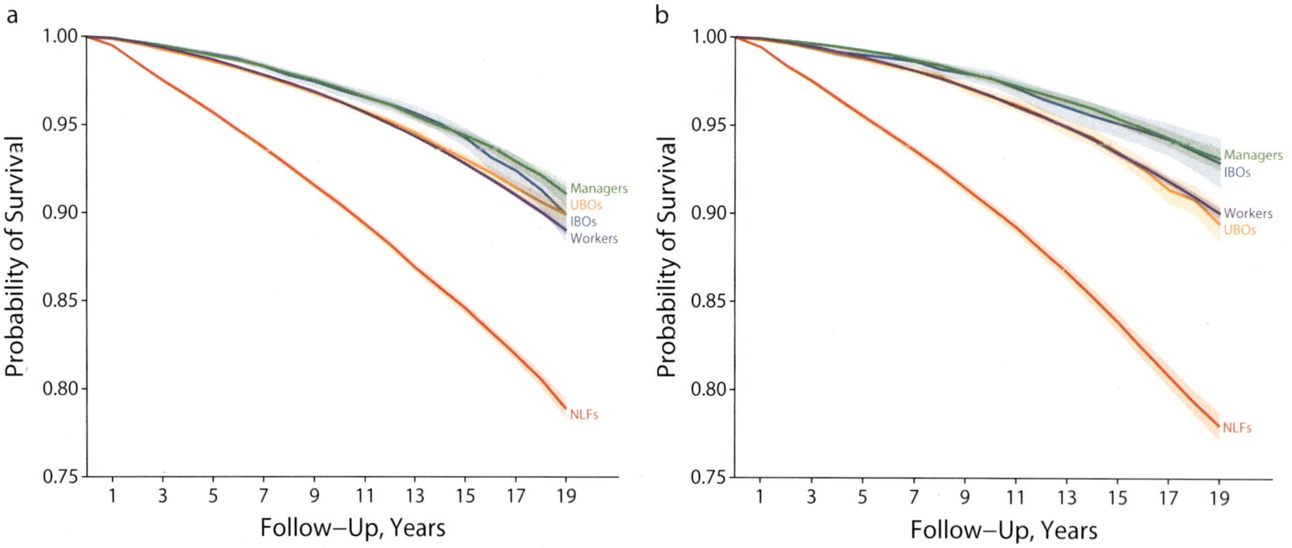

FIGURE 2— **Inverse-Probability-Weighted Kaplan–Meier Survival Curves Depicting Probability of Survival During Follow-Up by Class in (a) 1986–1996 With Follow-Up Through 2004 and (b) 2001–2019 With Follow-Up Through 2019: United States**

Note. IBOs = incorporated business owners; NLFs = those not in the labor force; UBOs = unincorporated business owners. Curves in left panel (a) estimated on sample of respondents aged 25–64 years to the United States' 1986–1996 National Health Interview Survey (NHIS) with mortality follow-up through December 31, 2004 (n = 564 202). Curves in right panel (b) estimated on similar sample, but restricted to the 2001–2018 NHIS with mortality follow-up through December 31, 2019 (n = 347 648). Via inverse probability weighting, estimates from curves are nationally representative and adjusted for gender, age, and interview year. Ninety-five percent confidence bands estimated with robust standard errors.

interaction rather than period stratification, although estimates were imprecise (online Appendix A6).

We also estimated greater class mortality inequities among men than women (Figure 3 and Appendix A7, available as a supplement to the online version of this article at http://www.ajph.org). For example, among men, UBOs, workers, and NLFs had, respectively, 7.9 (95% CI = −9.9, −5.9), 8.0 (95% CI = −9.8, −6.3), and 26.9 (95% CI = −29.1, −24.8) per 100 lower 34-year survival rate than IBOs. Meanwhile, among women, UBOs, workers, and NLFs had, respectively, just 5.5 (95% CI = −8.4, −2.5), 6.2 (95% CI = −8.9, −3.6), and 15.6 (95% CI = −18.3, −12.9) per 100 lower 34-year survival rates than IBOs.

Likewise, we estimated greater class mortality inequities among racially

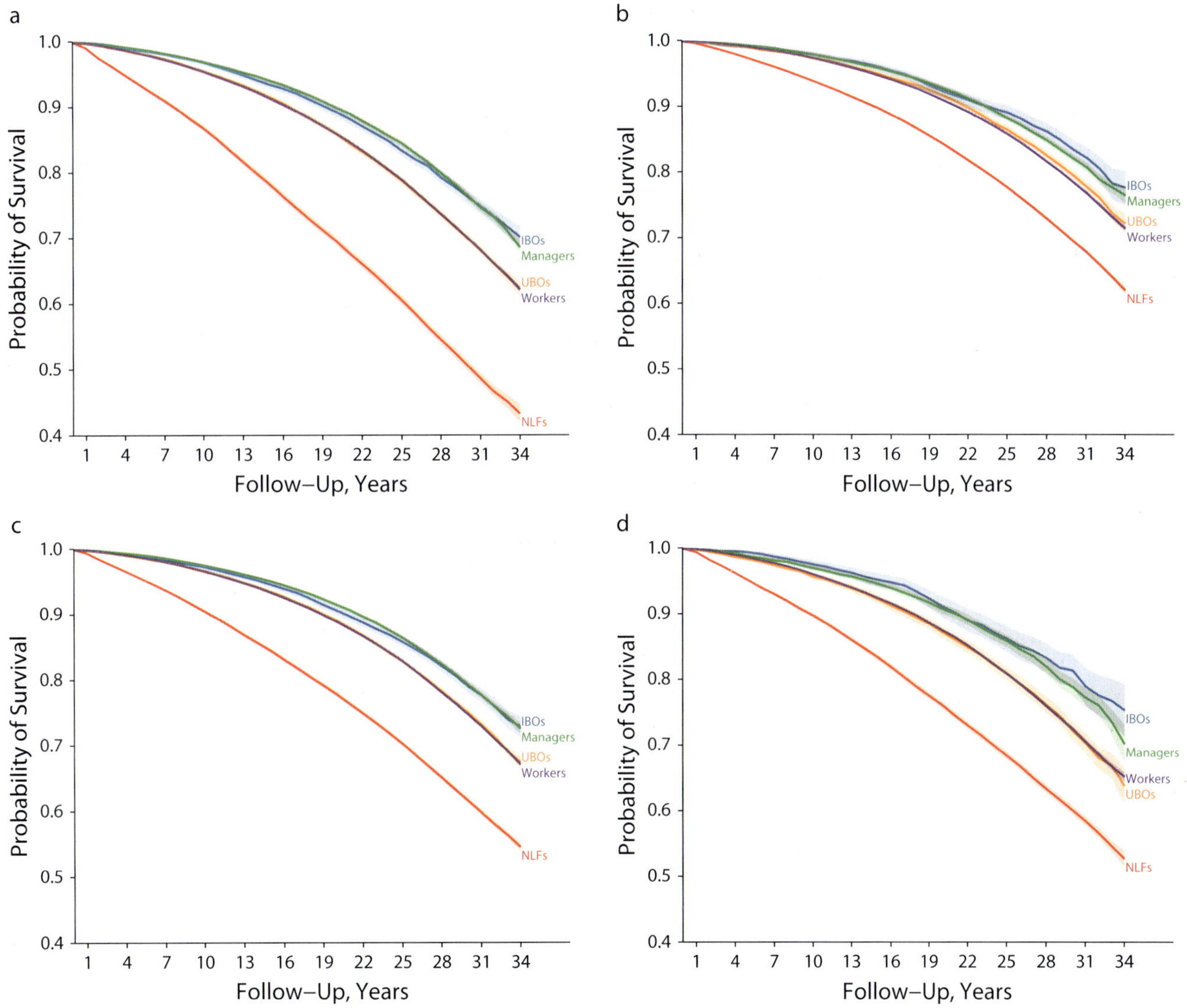

FIGURE 3— Inverse-Probability-Weighted Kaplan–Meier Survival Curves Depicting Probability of Survival During Follow-Up Among (a) Men, (b) Women, (c) Non-Hispanic White, and (d) Non-Hispanic Black, Hispanic, or Non-Hispanic Other: United States

Note. IBOs = incorporated business owners; NLFs = those not in the labor force; UBOs = unincorporated business owners. Curves estimated on sample of respondents aged 25–64 years to the United States' 1986–2018 National Health Interview Survey with mortality follow-up through December 31, 2019 (n = 911 850). Via inverse probability weighting, estimates from curves are nationally representative and adjusted for age and interview year. Class–race/ethnicity curves are additionally adjusted for gender. Ninety-five percent bands estimated with robust standard errors.

minoritized respondents than non-Hispanic White respondents (Figure 3 and Appendix A8, available as a supplement to the online version of this article at http://www.ajph.org). For example, among non-Hispanic Black, Hispanic, and non-Hispanic other respondents, UBOs, workers, and NLFs had, respectively, 11.5 (95% CI = −16.4, −6.7), 10.1 (95% CI = −14.2, −6.1), and 22.6 (95% CI = −26.8, −18.5) per 100 lower 34-year survival rates than IBOs. Meanwhile, among non-Hispanic White respondents, UBOs, workers, and NLFs had, respectively, just 5.4 (95% CI = −7.3, −3.5), 5.8 (95% CI = −7.5, −4.1), and 18.3 (95% CI = −20.1, −16.6) per 100 lower 34-year survival rates than IBOs. Racially minoritized IBOs had somewhat lower mortality risks than their non-Hispanic White counterparts, whereas racially minoritized UBOs, workers, and NLFs had somewhat higher mortality risks, fueling the group's elevated inequities.

Finally, we estimated greater class mortality inequities among less-educated than more-educated respondents (Appendix A9, available as a supplement to the online version of this article at http://www.ajph.org). For example, among those with a high school degree or less, UBOs, workers, and NLFs had, respectively, 5.7 (95% CI = −8.7, −2.7), 5.8 (95% CI = −8.6, −3.0), and 18.3 (95% CI = −21.2, −15.5) per 100 lower 34-year survival rates than IBOs. However, among those with more than a high school degree, UBOs, workers, and NLFs had, respectively, just 4.1 (95% CI = −6.3, −1.9), 3.3 (95% CI = −5.1, −1.4), and 13.1 (95% CI = −15.2, −11.1) per 100 lower 34-year survival rates than IBOs.

Cox models yielded substantively similar estimates to the curves (online Appendices A5–A9).

DISCUSSION

Using a relational social class measure based on power over property and labor, we analyzed the US class structure and class mortality inequities, including within time periods, genders, races/ethnicities, and educational groups.

We estimated that the class structure has remained mostly stable during the last 32 years, with workers constituting over half the population, including within genders and races/ethnicities. Nonetheless, women and racially minoritized respondents were segregated into the working class or excluded from the labor force entirely, whereas non-Hispanic White men were overrepresented among IBOs, UBOs, and managerial classes. These findings align with previous research[5,21] and suggest that labor-market segregation contributes to excess mortality among racially minoritized people.

We also estimated considerable class mortality inequities, with UBOs, NLFs, and workers (especially blue-collar, service, and unemployed workers) at greater mortality risk than IBOs and managers. The estimated inequities attenuated but persisted after adjustment for race/ethnicity, education, and other sociodemographics, suggesting—following European research on the topic[3]—that class inequities cannot be explained by different distributions of such factors across classes alone. We also estimated that class mortality inequities increased over time, driven by disproportionate mortality-rate decreases among managers and IBOs relative to changes among UBOs, workers, and NLFs. Such trends, which mirror trends in socioeconomic mortality inequities,[20] may partially reflect surging incomes among the upper classes relative to income changes among others,[19,34] an explanation that future research should investigate.

Finally, we estimated differences in class mortality inequities among sociodemographic subgroups, with greater inequities among male, racially minoritized, and less-educated respondents. Greater inequities among men may reflect a patriarchal gender division of labor, whereby economic well-being and health among heterosexual couples depend primarily on the man's class position and higher earnings.[15,35] Meanwhile, greater inequities among racially minoritized and less-educated respondents may reflect the segregation of marginalized workers and UBOs into especially oppressed segments of the class structure, including unemployment, hyperexploited service and blue-collar work, and precarious gig employment or sole proprietorship.[10–13] Moreover, such hazards may not be buffered by familial wealth or other resources available to the more privileged.[10]

Limitations

A primary limitation of our study is the NHIS's social class data. First, the NHIS lacks consistent data on whether respondents supervise anyone at work, a measure frequently used to distinguish workers from managers and the petite bourgeoisie from capitalists.[3] Given that we classified a lower proportion of respondents as "managers" than previous studies,[5,21] our "worker" subgroup likely contained respondents with supervisory authority who would have been classified as "managers" had the NHIS contained more detailed data. Moreover, those classified as "manager" were likely high-level managers with substantial authority and autonomy, including chief executives who share many characteristics with capitalists (e.g., stock options and delegated ownership authority). Second, we used incorporation status to distinguish business-owner subtypes. Although IBOs are more likely to employ workers than UBOs—making them more likely to be capitalists—many IBOs do not.[27] Thus, the owning classes in our study do not precisely coincide with the Marxist classes of "capitalists" and "petite bourgeoisie." Precise measurement would require consistent, detailed supervisory-authority data or data on the number of employees that employers employ, which are seldom available in epidemiological data sets.[3]

Another limitation is our coding of gender and race/ethnicity. First, interviewers generally assigned respondent gender—dichotomized as female and male—based on first name or relationship to household head. This assumes that gender is ascertainable from name and household structure alone, and may misclassify transgender, nonbinary, and other respondents, who face extensive labor-market discrimination.[9] Second, because of small counts, we could not subdivide "non-Hispanic Black," "Hispanic," and "non-Hispanic other" respondents in survival analyses. Such respondents experience unique forms of racism, including in the labor market.[12] Moreover, the class distribution varies across such subgroups, with non-Hispanic Black and Hispanic respondents less likely to be IBOs, UBOs, or managers than non-Hispanic "other" respondents (online Appendix 3). Thus, lumping these respondents together concealed probable mortality inequities.

Finally, the NHIS's income data are categorical, with only broad categories available in many years and changing top codes across waves, preventing us from quantifying how income disparities mediated class mortality inequities.

Despite these data limitations, the NHIS befitted our objectives, as it is among the largest, longest-running nationally representative epidemiological data sets containing detailed social class and mortality data.

Public Health Implications

We estimated considerable mortality inequities by class, gender, and race/ethnicity, inequities that may be increasing and that threaten population health. The COVID-19 pandemic has likely intensified the inequities, with harms concentrated among Black, Hispanic/Latinx, and Indigenous workers.[13] Our findings lay bare needs for structural interventions to build power among workers and other oppressed groups, including unionization campaigns, policies to strengthen labor protections and decommodify necessities, and social movements targeting broader economic transformation.[6] AJPH

ABOUT THE AUTHORS

Jerzy Eisenberg-Guyot and Megan C. Finsaas are with the Department of Epidemiology and Seth J. Prins is with the Departments of Epidemiology and Sociomedical Sciences, Mailman School of Public Health, Columbia University, New York, NY.

CORRESPONDENCE

Correspondence should be sent to Jerzy Eisenberg-Guyot, 722 West 168th St, 7th Fl, Room 720d, New York, NY 10032 (e-mail: je2433@cumc.columbia.edu). Reprints can be ordered at http://www.ajph.org by clicking the "Reprints" link.

PUBLICATION INFORMATION

Full Citation: Eisenberg-Guyot J, Finsaas MC, Prins SJ. Dead labor: mortality inequities by class, gender, and race/ethnicity in the United States, 1986–2019. *Am J Public Health*. 2023;113(6): 637–646.

Acceptance Date: January 3, 2023.

DOI: https://doi.org/10.2105/AJPH.2023.307227

CONTRIBUTORS

J. Eisenberg-Guyot conceptualized and designed the study, acquired the data, conducted the analyses, interpreted the results, and drafted the initial version of the article. The other authors advised J. Eisenberg-Guyot on study conceptualization, study design, and results interpretation, and provided feedback on subsequent drafts of the article. All authors approved the final version of the article and agree to be accountable for all aspects of the work.

ACKNOWLEDGMENTS

J. Eisenberg-Guyot's and M. C. Finsaas's research was supported by a grant from the National Institute of Mental Health of the National Institutes of Health (T32MH013043). S. J. Prins's research was supported by a grant from the National Institute on Drug Abuse of the National Institutes of Health (K01DA045955).

Note. The content of this article is solely the responsibility of the authors and does not represent the official position of the National Institutes of Health.

CONFLICTS OF INTEREST

The authors have no conflicts of interest to disclose.

HUMAN PARTICIPANT PROTECTION

This study used publicly available, deidentified data and thus was exempt from review by an institutional review board and informed consent requirements.

REFERENCES

1. Marx K. *Capital*. Vol I. London, UK: Penguin Classics; 1992.
2. Eisenberg-Guyot J, Prins SJ. The impact of capitalism on mental health: an epidemiological perspective. In: Bhugra D, Moussaoui D, Craig TJ, eds. *Oxford Textbook of Social Psychiatry*. New York, NY: Oxford University Press; 2022:195–204. Oxford Textbooks in Psychiatry series.
3. Muntaner C, Ng E, Chung H, Prins SJ. Two decades of neo-Marxist class analysis and health inequalities: a critical reconstruction. *Soc Theory Health*. 2015;13(3-4):267–287. https://doi.org/10.1057/sth.2015.17
4. Wright EO. *Class Counts: Comparative Studies in Class Analysis*. New York, NY: Cambridge University Press; 1997.
5. Eisenberg-Guyot J, Prins SJ, Muntaner C. Free agents or cogs in the machine? Classed, gendered, and racialized inequities in hazardous working conditions. *Am J Ind Med*. 2022;65(2): 92–104. https://doi.org/10.1002/ajim.23314
6. Harvey M. The political economy of health: revisiting its Marxian origins to address 21st-century health inequalities. *Am J Public Health*. 2021;111(2): 293–300. https://doi.org/10.2105/AJPH.2020.305996
7. Prins SJ, Bates LM, Keyes KM, Muntaner C. Anxious? Depressed? You might be suffering from

capitalism: contradictory class locations and the prevalence of depression and anxiety in the USA. *Sociol Health Illn.* 2015;37(8):1352–1372. https://doi.org/10.1111/1467-9566.12315

8. Eisenberg-Guyot J, Hajat A. Under capital's thumb: longitudinal associations between relational social class and health. *J Epidemiol Community Health.* 2020;74(5):453–459. https://doi.org/10.1136/jech-2019-213440
9. Krieger N. Measures of racism, sexism, heterosexism, and gender binarism for health equity research: from structural injustice to embodied harm—an ecosocial analysis. *Annu Rev Public Health.* 2020;41(1):37–62. https://doi.org/10.1146/annurev-publhealth-040119-094017
10. Bailey ZD, Krieger N, Agénor M, Graves J, Linos N, Bassett MT. Structural racism and health inequities in the USA: evidence and interventions. *Lancet.* 2017;389(10077):1453–1463. https://doi.org/10.1016/S0140-6736(17)30569-X
11. Laster Pirtle WN. Racial capitalism: a fundamental cause of novel coronavirus (COVID-19) pandemic inequities in the United States. *Health Educ Behav.* 2020;47(4):504–508. https://doi.org/10.1177/1090198120922942
12. Gee GC, Ford CL. Structural racism and health inequities: old issues, new directions. *Du Bois Rev.* 2011;8(1):115–132. https://doi.org/10.1017/S1742058X11000130
13. McClure ES, Vasudevan P, Bailey Z, Patel S, Robinson WR. Racial capitalism within public health: how occupational settings drive COVID-19 disparities. *Am J Epidemiol.* 2020;189(11):1244–1253. https://doi.org/10.1093/aje/kwaa126
14. Braverman H. The structure of the working class and its reserve armies. In: *Labor and Monopoly Capital.* New York, NY: Monthly Review Press; 1998:261–278.
15. Ferguson A, Hennessy R, Nagel M. Feminist perspectives on class and work. In: Zalta EN, ed. *The Stanford Encyclopedia of Philosophy.* Spring 2019. Metaphysics Research Lab, Stanford University. Available at: https://plato.stanford.edu/archives/spr2019/entries/feminism-class. Accessed June 27, 2020.
16. Brown H. Union Membership Byte 2021. Center for Economic and Policy Research. January 25, 2021. Available at: https://cepr.net/union-2021. Accessed August 10, 2022.
17. Malinowski B, Minkler M, Stock L. Labor unions: a public health institution. *Am J Public Health.* 2015;105(2):261–271. https://doi.org/10.2105/AJPH.2014.302309
18. Landsbergis PA, Choi B, Dobson M, et al. The key role of work in population health inequities. *Am J Public Health.* 2018;108(3):296–297. https://doi.org/10.2105/AJPH.2017.304288
19. Piketty T, Saez E, Zucman G. Distributional national accounts: methods and estimates for the United States. *Q J Econ.* 2018;133(2):553–609. https://doi.org/10.1093/qje/qjx043
20. Bosworth B. Increasing disparities in mortality by socioeconomic status. *Annu Rev Public Health.* 2018;39(1):237–251. https://doi.org/10.1146/annurev-publhealth-040617-014615
21. Eisenberg-Guyot J, Prins SJ. Relational social class, self-rated health, and mortality in the United States. *Int J Health Serv.* 2020;50(1):7–20. https://doi.org/10.1177/0020731419886194
22. Muntaner C, Hadden WC, Kravets N. Social class, race/ethnicity and all-cause mortality in the US: longitudinal results from the 1986–1994 National Health Interview Survey. *Eur J Epidemiol.* 2004;19(8):777–784. https://doi.org/10.1023/B:EJEP.0000036569.39399.68
23. National Center for Health Statistics. 2018 National Health Interview Survey (NHIS). Public use data release: survey description. 2019. Available at: https://ftp.cdc.gov/pub/Health_Statistics/NCHS/Dataset_Documentation/NHIS/2018/srvydesc.pdf. Accessed August 10, 2022.
24. National Center for Health Statistics. The Linkage of National Center for Health Statistics Survey Data to the National Death Index—2019 Linked Mortality File (LMF): linkage methodology and analytic considerations. 2022. Available at: https://www.cdc.gov/nchs/data/datalinkage/2019ndi-linkage-methods-and-analytic-considerations-508.pdf. Accessed August 10, 2022.
25. Blewett LA, Drew JAR, King ML, Williams KC, Del Ponte N, Convey P. IPUMS Health Surveys: National Health Interview Survey, Version 7.1. IPUMS. 2021. Available at: https://nhis.ipums.org. Accessed August 10, 2022.
26. Barbeau EM, Krieger N, Soobader MJ. Working class matters: socioeconomic disadvantage, race/ethnicity, gender, and smoking in NHIS 2000. *Am J Public Health.* 2004;94(2):269–278. https://doi.org/10.2105/AJPH.94.2.269
27. Kochhar R. Three-in-ten US jobs are held by the self-employed and the workers they hire: hiring more prevalent among self-employed Asians, whites, and men. Pew Research Center. 2015. Available at: https://www.pewresearch.org/social-trends/2015/10/22/three-in-ten-u-s-jobs-are-held-by-the-self-employed-and-the-workers-they-hire. Accessed August 11, 2022.
28. Christnacht CE, Smith A, Chenevert R. Measuring entrepreneurship in the American Community Survey: a demographic and occupational profile of self-employed workers. US Census Bureau. 2018. Available at: https://www.census.gov/content/dam/Census/library/working-papers/2018/demo/SEHSD-WP2018-28.pdf. Accessed August 11, 2022.
29. Austin PC. The use of propensity score methods with survival or time-to-event outcomes: reporting measures of effect similar to those used in randomized experiments. *Stat Med.* 2014;33(7):1242–1258. https://doi.org/10.1002/sim.5984
30. Geskus RB, van der Wal WM. R package "ipw" (version 1.0-11). 2015. Available at: https://cran.r-project.org/package=ipw. Accessed August 11, 2021.
31. Ridgeway G, Kovalchik SA, Griffin BA, Kabeto MU. Propensity score analysis with survey weighted data. *J Causal Inference.* 2015;3(2):237–249. https://doi.org/10.1515/jci-2014-0039
32. Therneau TM. R package "survival" (version 3.4-0). 2022. Available at: https://cran.r-project.org/package=survival. Accessed August 11, 2022.
33. Altman DG. Interaction revisited: the difference between two estimates. *BMJ.* 2003;326(7382):219. https://doi.org/10.1136/bmj.326.7382.219
34. Smith M, Yagan D, Zidar O, Zwick E. Capitalists in the twenty-first century. *Q J Econ.* 2019;134(4):1675–1745. https://doi.org/10.1093/qje/qjz020
35. Weeden KA, Cha Y, Bucca M. Long work hours, part-time work, and trends in the gender gap in pay, the motherhood wage penalty, and the fatherhood wage premium. *RSF Russell Sage Found J Soc Sci.* 2016;2(4):71–102. https://doi.org/10.7758/rsf.2016.2.4.03

COVID-19 Risk by Workers' Occupation and Industry in the United States, 2020–2021

Adam Gaffney, MD, MPH, David U. Himmelstein, MD, Danny McCormick, MD, MPH, and Steffie Woolhandler, MD, MPH

See also Hawkins, p. 631 and Leigh, p. 634.

Objectives. To assess the risk of COVID-19 by occupation and industry in the United States.

Methods. Using the 2020–2021 National Health Interview Survey, we estimated the risk of having had a diagnosis of COVID-19 by workers' industry and occupation, with and without adjustment for confounders. We also examined COVID-19 period prevalence by the number of workers in a household.

Results. Relative to workers in other industries and occupations, those in the industry "health care and social assistance" (adjusted prevalence ratio = 1.23; 95% confidence interval = 1.11, 1.37), or in the occupations "health practitioners and technical," "health care support," or "protective services" had elevated risks of COVID-19. However, compared with nonworkers, workers in 12 of 21 industries and 11 of 23 occupations (e.g., manufacturing, food preparation, and sales) were at elevated risk. COVID-19 prevalence rose with each additional worker in a household.

Conclusions. Workers in several industries and occupations with public-facing roles and adults in households with multiple workers had elevated risk of COVID-19.

Public Health Implications. Stronger workplace protections, paid sick leave, and better health care access might mitigate working families' risks from this and future pandemics. (*Am J Public Health.* 2023;113(6):647–656. https://doi.org/10.2105/AJPH.2023.307249)

AJPH June 2023, Vol 113, No. 6

The workplace has been recognized as a site of severe acute respiratory syndrome coronavirus 2 (SARS-CoV-2) transmission since the beginning of the pandemic.[1] In the United States, this prompted workplace closures, as well as telework for tens of millions of people beginning in March 2020.[2] However, many "essential" workers remained in the workplace or returned to in-person work in the first year of the pandemic: by October 2020, more than 100 million—disproportionately Black, Hispanic, and low-income US persons—were back in the workplace.[2] However, no comprehensive national COVID-19 workplace safety standard was implemented, and a vaccination or masking-plus-testing mandate for large employers proposed by the Occupational Safety and Health Administration (OSHA) was invalidated by the US Supreme Court.[3]

The extent to which workplace exposure led to population-level differences in COVID-19 incidence in the United States remains uncertain. Some population-level studies have identified differences in COVID-19 mortality by workers' occupation and industry in specific US workplaces, locales, and states. One found that workers in the transportation, material-moving, and health care–support occupations were at elevated risk of COVID-19 death in Massachusetts.[4] Another found notable increases in COVID-19 deaths among essential workers in California,[5,6] findings confirmed by a study that ascertained occupation using California state employment records.[7] Most recently, a Centers for Disease Control and Prevention (CDC) report found that, in 2020, COVID-19 mortality varied by industry and occupation across 46 states.[8] However, disparities in mortality—or in severe illness[9]—may reflect differences in health status or living conditions (e.g., household crowding) rather than workplace-related differences in COVID-19 exposure and infection.

Analyses of COVID-19 incidence that adjust for confounders such as household crowding may better isolate the effect of the workplace. For instance, a survey from the United Kingdom that used population-based sampling and testing found elevated risks for some occupational sectors (e.g., social care and protective services), even with adjustment for individual-level confounders.[10] However, fewer studies have examined population-level COVID-19 incidence by occupation and industry in the United States. An exception is a Wisconsin study that used state-collected occupational data ascertained during case investigations, which found the highest incidence of COVID-19 in personal care and service occupations, although occupation data were missing for 40% of cases.[11]

Reliable national US estimates of COVID-19 prevalence by occupation and industry are lacking, as well as information on whether the work status of 1 household member increases COVID-19 risk among other household members.

METHODS

We analyzed the 2020 and 2021 National Health Interview Survey (NHIS), a household survey conducted annually by the CDC. Although the NHIS usually interviews respondents in person in their homes, it interviewed many respondents by telephone during 2020 and 2021, when household response rates were 50.7% and 52.8% of those eligible, respectively. The NHIS collects detailed information on 1 randomly selected "sample adult" and "sample child" from each responding family.

We analyzed "sample adults" (aged ≥ 18 years) interviewed from quarter 3 of 2020 (when questions about COVID-19 were first asked) through quarter 4 of 2021. We focused on "workers" (i.e., adults working within the past year, defined by NHIS as those "who were working at or were on temporary leave from a paid job or business last week; or who worked, but not for pay at a family-owned job or business; or who did not have a job or business last week but had a job or business in the past 12 months"). This group included all seasonal and contract workers in 2020, but only those seasonal and contract workers working within the past 12 months in 2021.

For supplementary analyses, described herein, we also examined nonworking adults.

Variables

Exposures. Our main exposures were occupation and industry. NHIS provides detailed 2017 North American Industry Classification System codes for each worker (which it groups into 21 major sectors) and detailed 2018 Standard Occupational Classification codes (grouped into 23 major categories). Specific industries and occupations included in each category are available from the Census Bureau.[12] We used major sectors or categories for both industry and occupation because sample size precluded use of the more granular classifications. We excluded 608 respondents (2% of n = 28 875 workers) with missing data on industry or occupation (Appendix Figure A, available as a supplement to the online version of this article at https://ajph.org).

For some supplementary analyses, we included "non-workers" (defined as those aged > 17 years who were not "workers") and (in some statistical analyses) assigned them to a separate industry or occupation category ("no industry" and "no occupation," respectively).

In another supplementary analysis, we examined an additional exposure: the number of working adults in the household (0, 1, 2, or ≥ 3).

Outcome. Our outcome was having had COVID-19 at any time (i.e., answering yes to: "Has a doctor or other health professional ever told you that you had or likely had coronavirus or COVID-19?"); we excluded 265 observations (< 1% of sample) with missing or invalid responses (Appendix Figure A). Another question ascertained results of any COVID-19 testing, and those who reported a positive test were also defined as having had COVID-19. Approximately 90% of those who reported having had COVID-19 also reported a positive test; 95% of those reporting a positive test also reported having had COVID-19.

Analysis

We first examined workers' demographic characteristics (including age, gender, household size, and family income) by industry and occupation; we also calculated the proportion of each group that had at least 1 COVID-19 test.

Next, we calculated COVID-19 rates by workers' industry and occupation and among all workers and all nonworkers. We then performed Poisson regressions, unadjusted and adjusted, to examine the risk (period prevalence) of COVID-19 for workers in each industry and occupation relative to workers in all other industries and occupations. Poisson regressions estimate prevalence ratios (PRs) for binary outcomes.[13] We calculated standard errors using robust variance estimators.[13]

Our multivariable modeling approach[14] drew on previous studies of occupational COVID-19 risk,[9,15] other occupational hazards,[16] and biological plausibility.[17] Our aim was to isolate workplace exposures from other socioenvironmental factors likely to influence COVID-19 exposure. We selected covariates causally linked with COVID-19 infection risk (not disease severity) and employment, including age (18–24, 25–34, 35–44, 45–54, 55–64, and ≥ 65 years) and gender (male, female), both linked to COVID-19 risk in previous studies.[18,19] As a metric of household crowding, another risk factor for COVID-19 exposure,[20,21] we included household size (1, 2, 3, 4, 5, and ≥ 6 household members, calculated by summing the number of child and adult household members, each of which NHIS top-codes at 3). Finally, because income[22–24] may affect individuals' ability to avoid exposure (e.g., in shops or public transportation) irrespective of the work that produces this income, we included family income category relative to the federal poverty level according to US Census Bureau thresholds (< 100%, 100%–199%, 200%–299%, 300%–399%, 400%–499%, and ≥ 500%). We also performed sensitivity analyses using a parsimonious model (age- and gender-adjusted only).

Our multivariable regressions excluded individuals with missing data on covariates (n = 38 missing age; n = 55 missing household size; n = 3 missing gender).

Finally, we performed 2 sets of supplementary analyses. The first set examined COVID-19 risk among adults by industry and occupation (and all workers) but treated "no industry" and "no occupation" (i.e., nonworking adults) as the reference category. The second set examined COVID-19 risk but with the exposure redefined as the number of workers in the household; although this number is collinear with household size, our models included both variables to explore the independent effects of workplace exposure and household crowding.

We used NHIS-provided weights to generate national estimates and Stata/SE version 17 (Stata Corp LP, College Station, TX) survey procedures appropriate for complex sampling design; we used the COEFPLOT package for preparing figures.

RESULTS

Our primary analyses included 28 267 workers. Supplementary analyses additionally included 18 054 nonworking adults (Appendix Figure A).

Appendix Tables A and B provide demographic characteristics of workers by industry and occupation. Mean age ranged from 34 to 48 years across industries and occupations. The industry and occupation with the highest proportion of female workers was "health care and social assistance" (79.1%) and "personal care and service" (79.9%), respectively; the industry and occupation with the lowest proportion of female workers was "construction" (10.7%) and "construction/extraction" (3.7%), respectively. Household size averaged approximately 3 across industries and occupations, although race/ethnicity differed across industries and occupations. For example, only 1.9% and 11.6% of workers in the industry "management of companies and enterprises" were non-Hispanic Black or Hispanic, respectively. By contrast, 21.7% of workers in the "transportation and warehousing" industry were non-Hispanic Black, and 22.1% were Hispanic. From 50% to 70% of workers in most industries and occupations had at least 1 COVID-19 test.

Risk by Industry

Figure 1 provides the percentage of workers who had COVID-19 in each industry, as well as for all workers and nonworkers. Overall, 12.4% of workers versus 8.1% of nonworkers had experienced COVID-19; the adjusted percentages (data not shown) were 11.7% versus 9.1% (adjusted incidence ratio = 1.29; 95% confidence interval [CI] = 1.17, 1.41). The 5 industries with the highest proportion of workers experiencing COVID-19 were "health care and social assistance" (15.2%), "utilities" (14.8%), "wholesale trade" (14.5%), "manufacturing" (13.3%), and "accommodation and food services" (13.2%). The 5 industries with the lowest COVID-19 rates were the "armed forces" (6.9%), "management of companies and enterprises" (7.1%), "agriculture, forestry, fishing, and hunting" (7.1%), "information" (8.1%), and "professional, scientific, and technical services" (8.6%).

Appendix Figure A provides unadjusted and adjusted PRs of COVID-19 for each industry, with workers in all other industries treated as the reference group. Workers in 3 industries had a significantly reduced risk for COVID-19: "agriculture, forestry, fishing, and hunting" (adjusted PR [APR] = 0.59; 95% CI = 0.37, 0.96); "information" (APR = 0.67; 95% CI = 0.49, 0.91); and "professional, scientific and technical services" (APR = 0.74; 95% CI = 0.64, 0.87) industries. Only 1 industry, "health care and social assistance," had a significantly increased risk of COVID-19 compared with other industries (APR = 1.23; 95% CI = 1.11, 1.37). A model adjusted only for age and gender produced similar results (Appendix Figure B).

When the reference group was nonworkers (Appendix Figure C), workers in 12 of 21 industries had significantly higher adjusted risks of COVID-19 (e.g., "utilities" [APR = 1.66; 95% CI = 1.12, 2.47], "wholesale trade" [APR = 1.56; 95% CI = 1.17, 2.07], and "manufacturing" [APR = 1.42; 95% CI = 1.22, 1.65]).

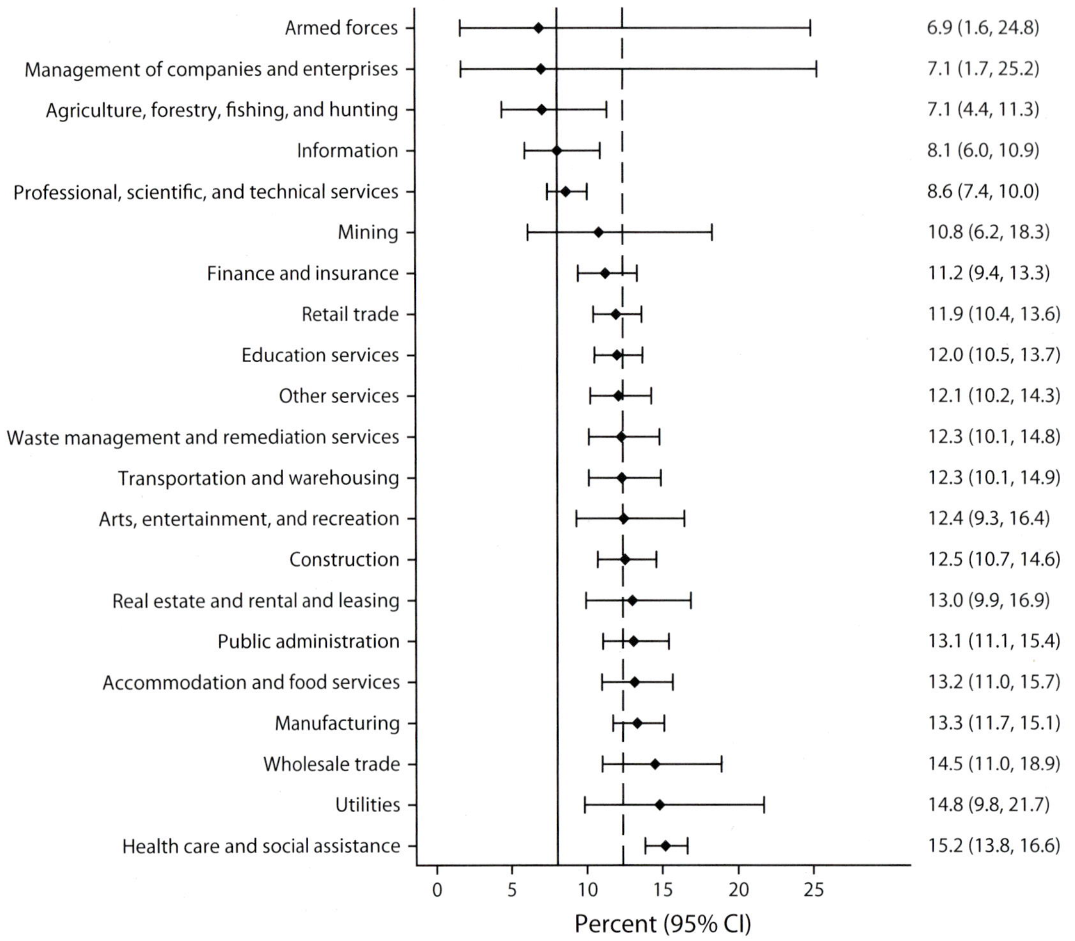

FIGURE 1— Percentage of Workers With COVID-19 by Industry: National Health Interview Survey, United States, 2020–2021

Note. CI = confidence interval. Sample size was n = 28 267. The solid vertical line indicates average COVID-19 infection rate among nonworkers. The dashed vertical line indicates COVID-19 infection rate among all workers. The full description for "waste management and remediation services" is "administrative and support and waste management and remediation services."

Risk by Occupation

Figure 2 provides COVID-19 rates by occupation. The occupations with the lowest COVID-19 risk were "legal" (5.2%; 95% CI = 3.3%, 8.3%), "life, physical, and social science" (5.6%; 95% CI = 3.5%, 8.8%), "military specific" (6.92%; 95% CI = 1.6%, 24.8%); "computer and mathematical" (8.7%; 95% CI = 7.0%, 10.8%); and "farming, fishing, and forestry occupations" (9.5%; 95% CI = 5.7%, 15.5%). The highest COVID-19 rates were in "protective services" (17.4%; 95% CI = 13.3%, 22.4%), "healthcare support" (16.9%; 95% CI = 14.1%, 20.1%), "community and social service" (15.1%; 95% CI = 11.7%, 19.3%), "healthcare practitioners and technical" (15.0%; 95% CI = 13.2%, 17.0%), and "food preparation and serving related" (14.9%; 95% CI = 12.2%, 18.0%) occupations.

Figure 3 shows results of unadjusted and adjusted regressions. Compared with all other occupations, 3—"legal" (APR = 0.47; 95% CI = 0.29, 0.76), "life/physical/social science" (APR = 0.47; 95% CI = 0.30, 0.75), and "computer and mathematical" (APR = 0.75; 95% CI = 0.60, 0.94)—had lower adjusted risk of COVID-19. Three occupations—"healthcare practitioners and technical" (APR = 1.23; 95% CI = 1.08, 1.41), "healthcare support" (APR = 1.26; 95% CI = 1.04, 1.53), and "protective services" (APR = 1.45; 95% CI = 1.11, 1.88)—had higher risk. Adjustment for only age and gender produced similar results (Appendix Figure D).

However, relative to nonworkers (Appendix Figure E), 11 of 23 occupations had an increased adjusted risk of COVID-19 (e.g., "food preparation and serving related" [APR = 1.37; 95%

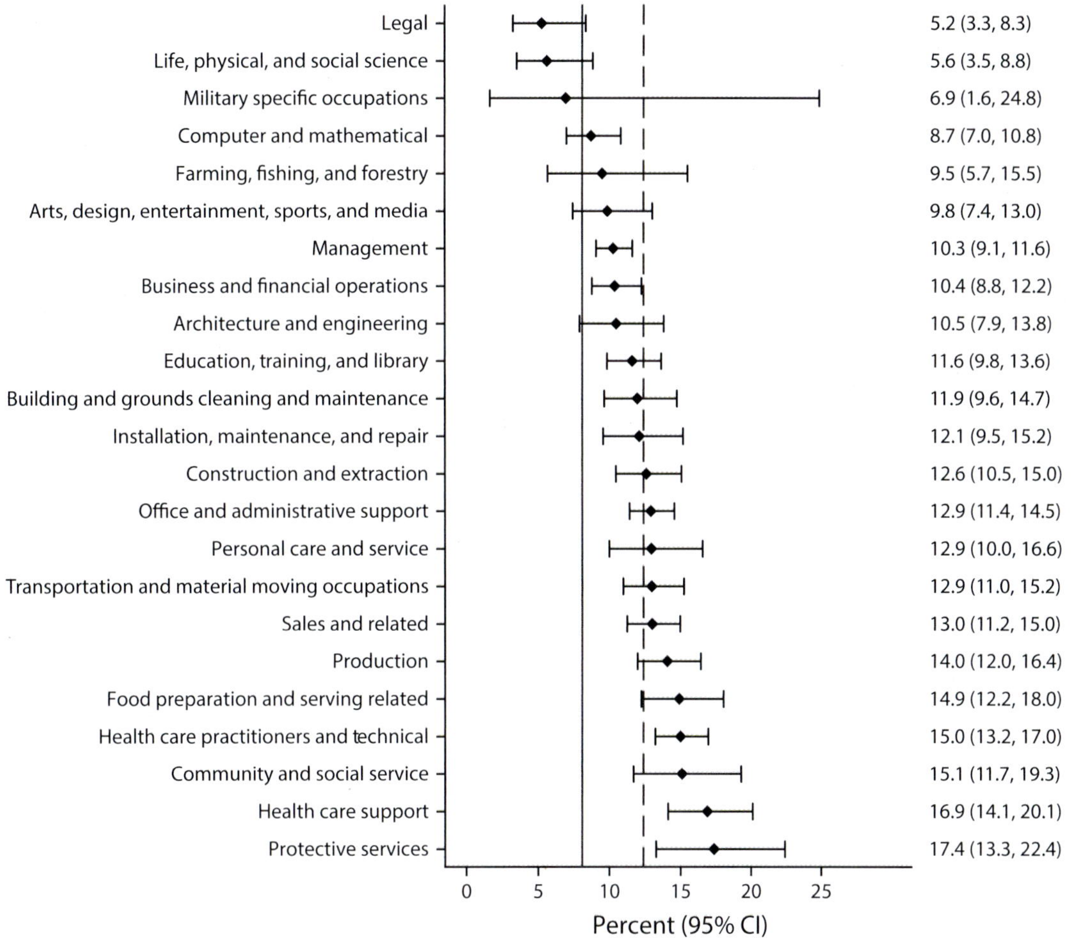

FIGURE 2— Percentage of Workers With COVID-19 by Occupation: National Health Interview Survey, United States, 2020–2021

Note. CI = confidence interval. Sample size was n = 28 267. The solid vertical line indicates average COVID-19 infection rate among nonworkers. The dashed vertical line indicates COVID-19 infection rate among all workers.

CI = 1.11, 1.68], "production" [APR = 1.42; 95% CI = 1.18, 1.71], and "sales and related" [APR = 1.32; 95% CI = 1.13, 1.54]).

Risk by Number of Workers in Household

Figure 4 provides the unadjusted and adjusted PRs for COVID-19 by the number of working adults in the household, showing a positive association. Compared with adults in households with no workers, those in households with 1 worker had an unadjusted COVID-19 PR of 1.49 (95% CI = 1.36, 1.65), with 2 workers a PR of 1.73 (95% CI = 1.59, 1.89), and with 3 or more workers a PR of 2.24 (95% CI = 1.97, 2.54). Multivariable adjustment, including for the total number of household adults, modestly attenuated these PRs.

DISCUSSION

In this analysis of nationally representative data, workers in the "health care and social assistance" industry (e.g., in hospitals, nursing homes, and practitioners' offices) had elevated COVID-19 risks relative to other workers, as did workers whose occupations were "healthcare support" (e.g., home health aides and nursing assistants), "protective services" (e.g., police officers, correctional officers, and school bus monitors), and "healthcare practitioners and technical occupations" (e.g., physicians, registered nurses, and emergency medical technicians). However, when compared with nonworkers, workers in multiple additional industries and occupations that generally require in-person or public-facing work—such as manufacturing, wholesale trade, food preparation, production, and sales—had increased

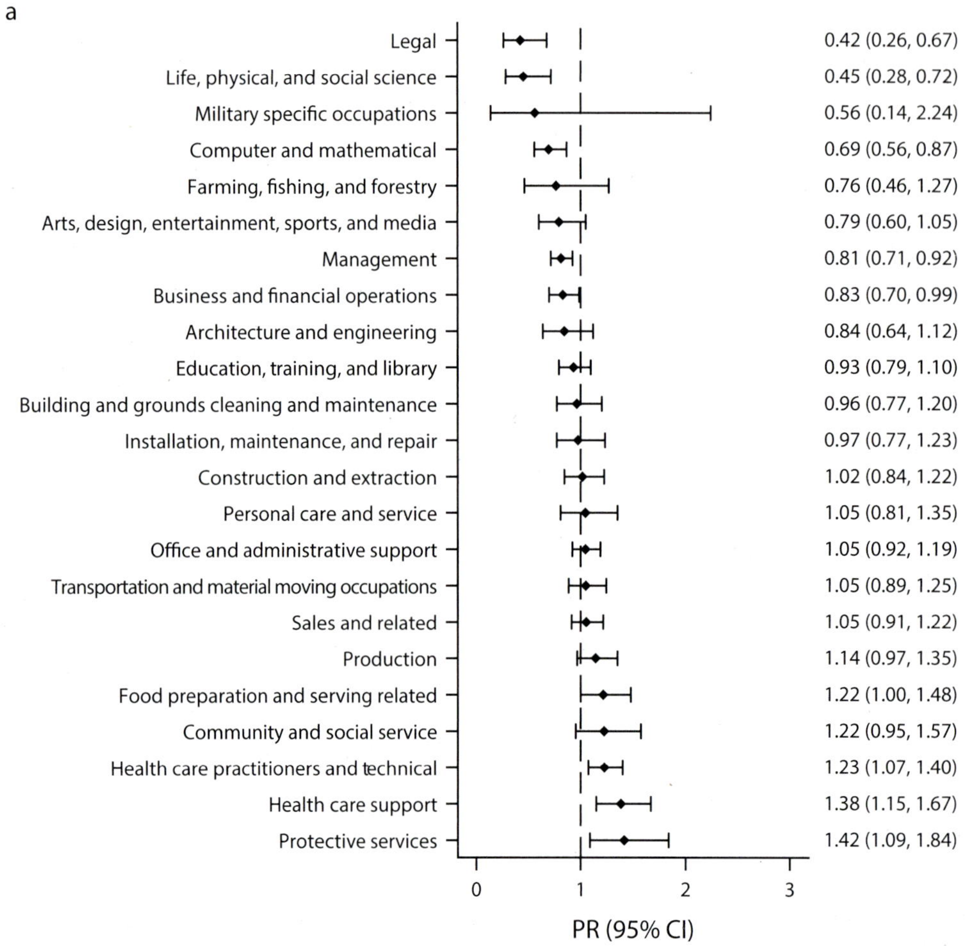

FIGURE 3— Risk of COVID-19 Diagnosis by Occupation (a) Unadjusted and (b) Adjusted: National Health Interview Survey, United States, 2020–2021

Note. CI = confidence interval; PR = prevalence ratio. Adjusted for age (18–24, 25–34, 35–44, 45–54, 55–64, and ≥ 65 years), gender (male, female), household size (1, 2, 3, 4, 5, and ≥ 6), and family income (< 100%, 100%–199%, 200%–299%, 300%–399%, 400%–499%, and ≥ 500% of federal poverty level according to US Census Bureau thresholds). Sample size for adjusted analyses was n = 28 172. The reference group for all prevalence ratios is adults working in all other occupations, indicated by the dashed vertical line.

COVID-19 risk, even with adjustment for age, gender, income, and household size. Notably, COVID-19 risk also rose with each additional worker within a household. These findings provide further, nationally representative evidence of differential risk of occupational COVID-19 infection, including for some health care personnel (e.g., practitioners) with relatively high incomes and status.

Workplace-based outbreaks of SARS-CoV-2 infection have been described since the outset of the pandemic, including in health care settings in Wuhan, China—leading 1 observer to call COVID-19 "the first new occupational disease . . . in this decade."[1] Even before the pandemic, however, workplaces were known to play an important role in viral transmission. Influenza studies, for instance, have suggested that a substantial proportion of interpersonal contacts and transmission occurs at work.[25] While many earlier COVID-19 studies focused on health care workers,[26] a growing number have included other occupations and industries. However, most studies were unable to control for household size or income, key factors relating to risk of COVID-19.[20] A notable exception is a recent analysis of COVID-19 mortality in 14.3 million British adults, although occupation was assessed approximately a decade before the pandemic.[27]

Our finding of increased COVID-19 risk among US workers in on-site, public-facing employment expands on the previous literature in several respects. First, while many previous analyses have focused on specific workplaces[28] or states,[5–7,11,29] ours is

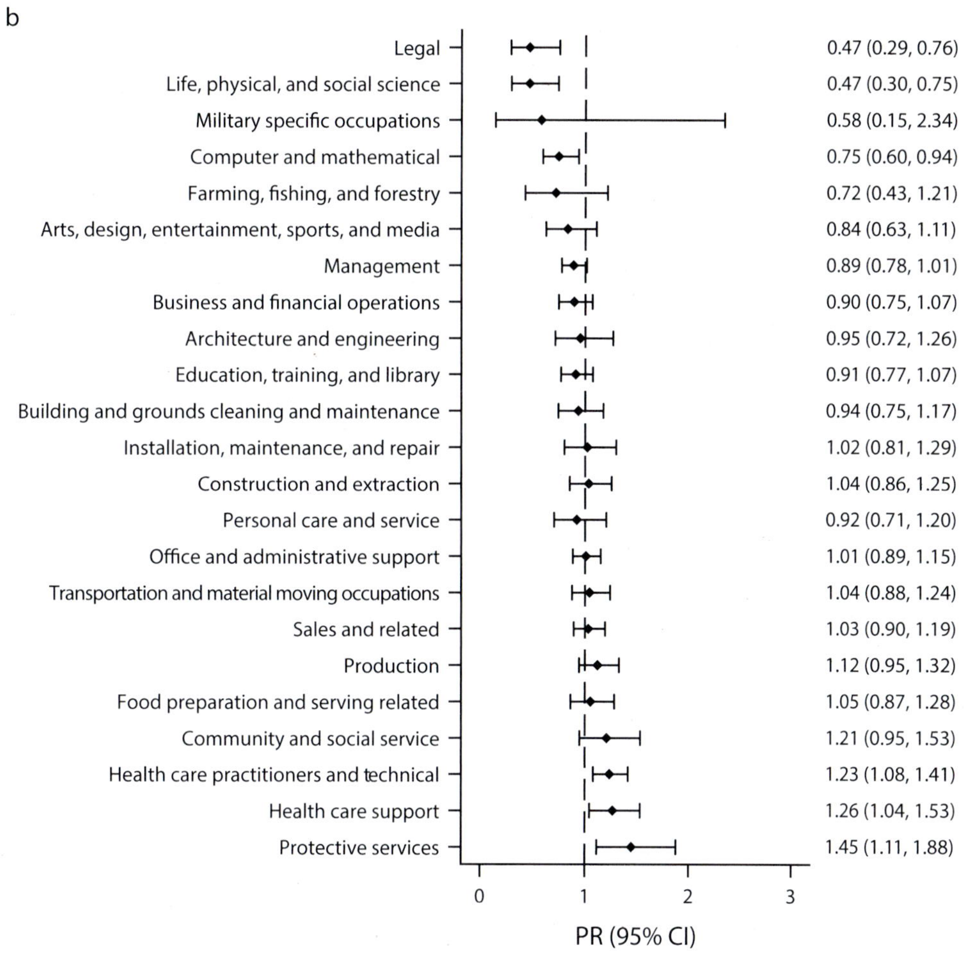

FIGURE 3— Continued

nationally representative. Second, our interview data permit more accurate assessment of occupation than all but 1[7] US death certificate–based analysis, which used California state employment records. Third, we were able to control for household size. Finally, we uniquely identified a linear relationship between the number of workers in a household and risk of COVID-19—underscoring that COVID-19 poses occupational risks not only for workers but also for those in their household.

Limitations

Our study has limitations. As with most analyses of COVID-19, we cannot determine where the infection was acquired. However, we controlled for important variables correlated with COVID-19 risk, including household size and income, although we lacked data on home characteristics, especially the number of rooms. In addition, we defined industry and occupation using respondents' current (or most recent) job but lacked data on the timing of COVID-19 diagnosis. Hence, some respondents may have changed their occupation (or industry) between their COVID-19 diagnosis and the interview, although the numbers are likely small given the short time frame encompassed by our data.

We also did not explore how occupational risks changed over time. In addition, the occupational and industry categories we used were quite broad; hence, our analysis could miss variability in risk between jobs within a category (e.g., between police officers and bus monitors). We had no data on teleworking, although we hypothesize that this is predicted by occupation and industry. In addition, differential rates of testing across industries and occupations could bias our findings, although the alignment of our findings with previous studies, as well as the consistency of our results with occupational exposure risk factors,[15,30] suggests that increased testing alone is unlikely to fully account

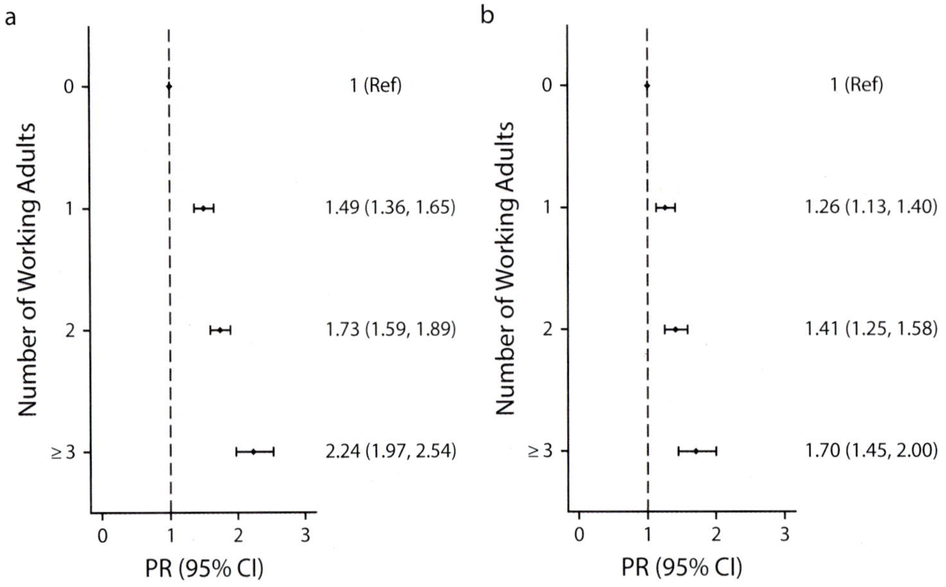

FIGURE 4— Risk of COVID-19 Diagnosis Among Adults by Number of Working Household Adults (a) Unadjusted and (b) Adjusted: National Health Interview Survey, United States, 2020–2021

Note. CI = confidence interval; PR = prevalence ratio. Sample size was n = 46 245. Adjusted for age (18–24, 25–34, 35–44, 45–54, 55–64, and ≥ 65 years), gender (male, female), household size (1, 2, 3, 4, 5, and ≥ 6), and family income (< 100%, 100%–199%, 200%–299%, 300%–399%, 400%–499%, and ≥ 500% of federal poverty level according to US Census Bureau thresholds). Sample size for adjusted analyses was n = 46 142.

for our findings. Our population excluded persons who died of COVID-19 before being interviewed; however, our findings were congruent with previous death certificate–based studies.

Finally, the choice of reference group affects interpretation of study results. Our comparison of workers in each industry or occupation to all other workers likely underestimates occupational risk (because the reference category also experiences some risk). Conversely, our comparisons of workers to nonworkers are subject to residual confounding and, hence, may overstate (or understate) occupational risk.

Public Health Implications

Early in the pandemic, the Trump administration met well-publicized occupational outbreaks, such as in meatpacking plants, with anemic regulatory responses.[31] The Office of the Inspector General found that, while complaints to OSHA rose in 2020 from the previous year, the number of inspections—most of which were conducted remotely—fell.[32] Meanwhile, the Office of the Inspector General noted that although OSHA had issued "guidance" on COVID-19 precautions, it had failed to issue an Emergency Temporary Standard to mandate stronger and more enforceable protections.[32]

In February 2021, President Biden issued an executive order directing OSHA to strengthen its COVID-19 protections. However, the national, comprehensive Emergency Temporary Standard that OSHA initially drafted[33] was ultimately narrowed to a standard for health care workers and, late in 2021, to one that would have primarily mandated vaccination (or masking plus testing) at large businesses. Even that narrower vaccination versus masking-plus-testing mandate, however, was stayed by legal challenge and then invalidated by the Supreme Court in January 2022.

Our and previous analyses suggest that the lack of adequate workplace protections during the COVID-19 pandemic worsened its toll. To reduce respiratory virus transmission, occupational safety standards are still needed. Such standards might include requirements for improved indoor air quality (i.e., specific benchmarks as recently proposed[34]), provision of personal protective equipment (e.g., high-quality masks), and vaccine mandates in some settings (e.g., health care facilities, or more broadly during severe surges).

More data on occupational risks of COVID-19 and systems for robust population-level respiratory viral surveillance could inform such policies; Britain's Office for National Statistics' COVID-19 serosurvey could serve as a model. In addition, universal social insurance, including paid sick leave (and assurance that using it will not incur retaliation), universal health care coverage and improved vaccine access, and workers' compensation for infectious diseases like COVID-19 could help mitigate the harms of workplace exposures during this and future pandemics. In very-high-mortality situations, however, keeping workers out of the workplace may be the safest approach, albeit one requiring ample social and economic support. AJPH

ABOUT THE AUTHORS

Adam Gaffney and Danny McCormick are with the Department of Medicine, Cambridge Health Alliance, Cambridge, MA, and Harvard Medical School, Boston, MA. David Himmelstein and Steffie Woolhandler are with City University of New York at Hunter College, New York, NY; Department of Medicine, Cambridge Health Alliance; Harvard Medical School; and Public Citizen Health Research Group, Washington, DC.

CORRESPONDENCE

Correspondence should be sent to Adam Gaffney, Cambridge Health Alliance, 1493 Cambridge St, Cambridge, MA 02139 (e-mail: agaffney@challiance.org). Reprints can be ordered at https://ajph.org by clicking the "Reprints" link.

PUBLICATION INFORMATION

Full Citation: Gaffney A, Himmelstein DU, McCormick D, Woolhandler S. COVID-19 risk by workers' occupation and industry in the United States, 2020–2021. *Am J Public Health*. 2023;113(6):647–656.

Acceptance Date: January 27, 2023.

DOI: https://doi.org/10.2105/AJPH.2023.307249

CONTRIBUTORS

All authors contributed to the concept and design of the study. A. Gaffney performed the analyses. All authors contributed to the interpretation of the data. All authors either participated in drafting the article or critically reviewed the article. All authors agree to publication of the final submitted version of the article.

CONFLICTS OF INTEREST

A. Gaffney is a past president of Physicians for a National Health Program, a nonprofit organization that favors coverage expansion through a single-payer program; he has not received any compensation from that group, although some of his travel on behalf of the organization was previously reimbursed by it. The spouse of A. Gaffney is an employee of Treatment Action Group, a nonprofit research and policy think tank focused on HIV, tuberculosis, and hepatitis C treatment.

HUMAN PARTICIPANT PROTECTION

Analyses of de-identified, public use data are not considered human participant research by the institutional review boards of the authors' institutions.

REFERENCES

1. Koh D. Occupational risks for COVID-19 infection. *Occup Med (Lond)*. 2020;70(1):3–5. https://doi.org/10.1093/occmed/kqaa036
2. Gaffney AW, Himmelstein DU, Woolhandler S. Trends and disparities in teleworking during the COVID-19 pandemic in the USA: May 2020–February 2021. *J Gen Intern Med*. 2021;36(11):3647–3649. https://doi.org/10.1007/s11606-021-07078-9
3. Michaels D, Barab J. Opinion. OSHA can do more to protect Americans from Covid-19. *New York Times*. January 15, 2022. Available at: https://www.nytimes.com/2022/01/14/opinion/supreme-court-vaccine-mandate-osha.html. Accessed September 29, 2022.
4. Hawkins D, Davis L, Kriebel D. COVID-19 deaths by occupation, Massachusetts, March 1–July 31, 2020. *Am J Ind Med*. 2021;64(4):238–244. https://doi.org/10.1002/ajim.23227
5. Chen YH, Glymour M, Riley A, et al. Excess mortality associated with the COVID-19 pandemic among Californians 18–65 years of age, by occupational sector and occupation: March through November 2020. *PLoS One*. 2021;16(6):e0252454. https://doi.org/10.1371/journal.pone.0252454
6. Chen YH, Riley AR, Duchowny KA, et al. COVID-19 mortality and excess mortality among working-age residents in California, USA, by occupational sector: a longitudinal cohort analysis of mortality surveillance data. *Lancet Public Health*. 2022;7(9):e744–e753. https://doi.org/10.1016/S2468-2667(22)00191-8
7. Cummings KJ, Beckman J, Frederick M, et al. Disparities in COVID-19 fatalities among working Californians. *PLoS One*. 2022;17(3):e0266058. https://doi.org/10.1371/journal.pone.0266058
8. Billock R, Steege A, Miniño A. COVID-19 mortality by usual occupation and industry: 46 states and New York City, United States, 2020. National Center for Health Statistics. July 2022. Available at: https://stacks.cdc.gov/view/cdc/120292. Accessed December 5, 2022.
9. Mutambudzi M, Niedwiedz C, Macdonald EB, et al. Occupation and risk of severe COVID-19: prospective cohort study of 120 075 UK Biobank participants. *Occup Environ Med*. 2020;78(5):307–314. https://doi.org/10.1136/oemed-2020-106731
10. Rhodes S, Wilkinson J, Pearce N, et al. Occupational differences in SARS-CoV-2 infection: analysis of the UK ONS COVID-19 infection survey. *J Epidemiol Community Health*. 2022;76(10):841–846. https://doi.org/10.1136/jech-2022-219101
11. Pray IW, Grajewski B, Morris C, Modji K, DeJonge P, McCoy K, et al. Measuring work-related risk of COVID-19: comparison of COVID-19 incidence by occupation and industry—Wisconsin, September 2020–May 2021. *Clin Infect Dis*. 2023;76(3):e163–e171. https://doi.org/10.1093/cid/ciac586
12. US Census Bureau. Industry and occupation code lists & crosswalks. Available at: https://www.census.gov/topics/employment/industry-occupation/guidance/code-lists.html. Accessed December 3, 2022.
13. Zou G. A modified Poisson regression approach to prospective studies with binary data. *Am J Epidemiol*. 2004;159(7):702–706. https://doi.org/10.1093/aje/kwh090
14. VanderWeele TJ. Principles of confounder selection. *Eur J Epidemiol*. 2019;34(3):211–219. https://doi.org/10.1007/s10654-019-00494-6
15. Baker MG, Peckham TK, Seixas NS. Estimating the burden of United States workers exposed to infection or disease: a key factor in containing risk of COVID-19 infection. *PLoS One*. 2020;15(4):e0232452. https://doi.org/10.1371/journal.pone.0232452
16. Krieger N, Chen JT, Waterman PD, et al. The inverse hazard law: blood pressure, sexual harassment, racial discrimination, workplace abuse and occupational exposures in US low-income Black, White and Latino workers. *Soc Sci Med*. 2008;67(12):1970–1981. https://doi.org/10.1016/j.socscimed.2008.09.039
17. Wilson AM, Sleeth DK, Schaefer C, Jones RM. Transmission of respiratory viral diseases to health care workers: COVID-19 as an example. *Annu Rev Public Health*. 2022;43(1):311–330. https://doi.org/10.1146/annurev-publhealth-052120-110009
18. Doerre A, Doblhammer G. The influence of gender on COVID-19 infections and mortality in Germany: insights from age- and gender-specific modeling of contact rates, infections, and deaths in the early phase of the pandemic. *PLoS One*. 2022;17(5):e0268119. https://doi.org/10.1371/journal.pone.0268119
19. Clarke KEN. Seroprevalence of infection-induced SARS-CoV-2 antibodies—United States, September 2021–February 2022. *MMWR Morb Mortal Wkly Rep*. 2022;71(17):606–608. https://doi.org/10.15585/mmwr.mm7117e3
20. Nash D, Qasmieh S, Robertson M, et al. Household factors and the risk of severe COVID-like illness early in the US pandemic. *PLoS One*. 2022;17(7):e0271786. https://doi.org/10.1371/journal.pone.0271786
21. Gouse I, Walters S, Miller-Archie S, Singh T, Lim S. The role of housing characteristics in racial and ethnic disparities in SARS-CoV-2 antibody seropositivity among New York City adults: a population representative study. *Prev Med*. 2022;164:107287. https://doi.org/10.1016/j.ypmed.2022.107287
22. Adams C, Horton M, Solomon O, et al. Health inequities in SARS-CoV-2 infection, seroprevalence, and COVID-19 vaccination: results from the East Bay COVID-19 study. *PLOS Global Public Health*. 2022;2(8):e0000647. https://doi.org/10.1371/journal.pgph.0000647
23. Karmakar M, Lantz PM, Tipirneni R. Association of social and demographic factors with COVID-19 incidence and death rates in the US. *JAMA Netw Open*. 2021;4(1):e2036462. https://doi.org/10.1001/jamanetworkopen.2020.36462
24. Tan AX, Hinman JA, Abdel Magid HS, Nelson LM, Odden MC. Association between income inequality and county-level COVID-19 cases and deaths in the US. *JAMA Netw Open*. 2021;4(5):e218799. https://doi.org/10.1001/jamanetworkopen.2021.8799

25. Edwards CH, Tomba GS, de Blasio BF. Influenza in workplaces: transmission, workers' adherence to sick leave advice and European sick leave recommendations. *Eur J Public Health.* 2016; 26(3):478–485. https://doi.org/10.1093/eurpub/ckw031
26. Chou R, Dana T, Buckley DI, Selph S, Fu R, Totten AM. Update alert 11: Epidemiology of and risk factors for coronavirus infection in health care workers. *Ann Intern Med.* 2022;175(8):W83–W84. https://doi.org/10.7326/L22-0235
27. Nafilyan V, Pawelek P, Ayoubkhani D, et al. Occupation and COVID-19 mortality in England: a national linked data study of 14.3 million adults. *Occup Environ Med.* 2022;79(7):433–441. https://doi.org/10.1136/oemed-2021-107818
28. Lan FY, Suharlim C, Kales SN, Yang J. Association between SARS-CoV-2 infection, exposure risk and mental health among a cohort of essential retail workers in the USA. *Occup Environ Med.* 2021;78(4):237–243. https://doi.org/10.1136/oemed-2020-106774
29. Hawkins D. Differential occupational risk for COVID-19 and other infection exposure according to race and ethnicity. *Am J Ind Med.* 2020; 63(9):817–820. https://doi.org/10.1002/ajim.23145
30. Zhang M. Estimation of differential occupational risk of COVID-19 by comparing risk factors with case data by occupational group. *Am J Ind Med.* 2021;64(1):39–47. https://doi.org/10.1002/ajim.23199
31. New report says failures at OSHA under Trump could have put more workers at risk during pandemic. *Washington Post.* March 2, 2021. Available at: http://www.washingtonpost.com/business/2021/03/02/osha-inspections-covid-oig-report. Accessed September 26, 2022.
32. Office of Inspector General, Office of Audit. COVID-19: increased worksite complaints and reduced OSHA inspections leave US workers' safety at increased risk. Department of Labor. February 25, 2021. Available at: https://www.oversight.gov/report/DOL/COVID-19-Increased-Worksite-Complaints-and-Reduced-OSHA-Inspections-Leave-US-Workers. Accessed September 26, 2022.
33. Rolfsen B. OSHA virus rule intended to cover all workers, draft shows (1). Bloomberg Law. June 28, 2021. Available at: https://news.bloomberglaw.com/safety/osha-covid-19-rule-intended-to-cover-all-workers-draft-shows. Accessed September 29, 2022.
34. The Lancet COVID-19 Commission Task Force on Safe Work, Safe School, and Safe Travel. Proposed non-infectious air delivery rates (NADR) for reducing exposure to airborne respiratory infectious diseases. November 2022. Available at: https://static1.squarespace.com/static/5ef3652ab722df11fcb2ba5d/t/637740d40f35a9699a7fb05f/1668759764821/Lancet+Covid+Commission+TF+Report+Nov+2022.pdf. Accessed December 3, 2022.

Excess Injury Mortality in Washington State During the 2021 Heat Wave

Joan A. Casey, PhD, MA, Robbie M. Parks, PhD, MA, Tim A. Bruckner, PhD, MPH, Alison Gemmill, PhD, MA, MPH, and Ralph Catalano, PhD, MRP

Objectives. To determine whether the 2021 Pacific Northwest heat wave resulted in excess injury (both unintentional and intentional) deaths.

Methods. With US death certificate data from December 29, 2013, to July 31, 2021, we generated weekly counts of injury deaths in Washington State and the rest of the country. We used time-series methods to identify excess injury deaths that may have occurred during and following the anomalously warm temperature period based on those expected from history and from simultaneous deaths in the remainder of the United States.

Results. Beginning the week including June 25, 2021 (heat wave initiation), 3 weeks exceeded the expected count of injury deaths in Washington State, with an estimated total of 159 excess injury deaths (95% detection interval = 122, 195) during the 3-week period.

Conclusions. The 2021 Pacific Northwest heat wave was associated with an increase in injury deaths.

Public Health Implications. Under global warming scenarios, heat waves of this magnitude will become much more common. Adaptation and planning efforts are needed to protect residents of the historically temperate Pacific Northwest for a range of health outcomes. (*Am J Public Health*. 2023;113(6): 657–660. https://doi.org/10.2105/AJPH.2023.307269)

AJPH June 2023, Vol 113, No. 6

Heat waves—extended periods of anomalously warm temperatures—are a critical public health concern, and a key driver for seeking adaptation measures against climate change.[1] Although assessments of the health effects of anomalously warm temperatures have largely focused on natural causes of deaths, including cardiorespiratory diseases and parasitic and infectious diseases, there is growing evidence of a robust association with deaths from injuries, such as from drownings, transport accidents, assaults, and suicides.[2–4] Previous work has also illustrated the risk of injury that heat poses among construction[5] and agricultural[6] workers in Washington State.

The Pacific Northwest region of the United States has a historically temperate climate. Late June and early July 2021, however, brought the highest temperatures ever recorded in the region.[7] Seattle, Washington, for example, experienced record heat on 3 consecutive days ending June 28, when temperatures peaked at 42°C, exceeding the previous recorded high by 3°C.[7] Attributed to climate change,[7] this period of anomalously warm temperatures centered on the Pacific Northwest, a region with minimal history of extreme heat events and thus relatively unprepared regarding infrastructure and prevalence of air conditioning.[8]

Such an anomalously warm temperature period may have induced excess injury deaths. Here, we define excess injury deaths as the difference between the observed number of injury deaths during a period of anomalously warm temperatures and a counterfactual scenario in which elevated temperatures had not occurred.[9] We estimate excess injury deaths, if any, during the anomalously warm temperature 2021 period, as the difference between injury deaths in Washington State expected from history and injury deaths in the rest of the United States at the same time as the heat wave.

METHODS

We used nationwide death certificate data from December 29, 2013, to July

31, 2021 (provisional at the time of analysis in December 2022). Death certificates in the United States use a "manner of death" classification, set by the Centers for Disease Control and Prevention, that includes "natural death," defined as "due solely or nearly totally to disease and/or the aging process." Based on data from 2010 to 2020, natural deaths accounted for approximately 89% of deaths in the United States.[10] We calculated the weekly count of Washington State injury deaths, also known as external or unnatural deaths, in the 396 study period weeks by subtracting natural from all-cause deaths.

We used time-series methods to determine whether the late June to early July 2021 heat wave in Washington State coincided with excess injury deaths. Our analyses, conducted using Scientific Computing Associates Software (Villa Park, IL), proceeded through the following steps:

1. We regressed the weekly count of injury deaths in Washington State on those in the remainder of the United States for the 390 weeks (i.e., December 29, 2013, through June 19, 2021) before the onset of the heat wave. This regression controlled determinants of temporal variation in injury death (e.g., long-term trends, seasonal trends, changes in death registration definitions and procedures) shared by Washington State and the rest of country.
2. We used Box–Jenkins methods to identify and model autocorrelation in the residuals of the step 1 regression. This step yielded a Box–Jenkins "transfer function" or equation that estimated Washington State injury deaths from those in the remainder of the United States and from autocorrelation specific to Washington State. Residuals of the transfer function satisfied the assumption of normal and independent distribution around 0.
3. We applied the Box–Jenkins transfer function devised in step 2, with coefficients fixed to those estimated for the first 390 weeks, to the full 396 weeks of observed data.
4. We combined the residuals from steps 1 and 3 and graphed them as well as the 95% detection interval of the residuals from step 1. We specified the lower and upper bounds of the detection interval as the negatively and positively signed product of 1.96 and the standard deviation of the residuals.

Because injury mortality (e.g., suicide) may lag exposure, and prior studies of heat and injury mortality relied on monthly data,[2,3] we evaluated excess injury mortality in the week of—and in the 5 weeks following—the heat wave. If the processes that yielded injury deaths in Washington State remained unaffected by the shock of the 2021 heat wave, the last 6 residuals (i.e., June–July 2021) in the graph produced in step 4 should have appeared randomly sampled from the prior 390 weeks. If, however, extreme ambient heat was associated with increased injury deaths, at least 1 of the last 6 residuals would rise above the 95% detection interval.

RESULTS

Between December 29, 2013, and June 19, 2021, weekly injury deaths in Washington State ranged from 56 to 154 (mean = 99; SD = 15). Figure 1 illustrates observed deaths throughout the study period, with noticeable upticks in injury deaths nationwide during the COVID-19 pandemic and in Washington State during the 2021 Pacific Northwest heat wave. As described in the Appendix (available as a supplement to the online version of this article at http://www.ajph.org), steps 1 and 2 produced a transfer function showing that weekly injury deaths in Washington State correlated with those nationwide. Time-series analyses found that injury death counts exceeded expected counts in the 3 weeks starting June 20 and ending July 10 (online Appendix, Figures A and B). During the week of June 20, injury deaths exceeded expected counts by 21 (1 injury death above the 95% detection interval of 20); during the week of record temperature (i.e., that ending July 3, 2021), injury deaths exceeded expected counts by 93 (72 injury deaths above the 95% detection interval of 20); and during the week beginning July 4, injury deaths exceeded expected counts by 45 (25 injury deaths above the 95% detection interval). We therefore estimated that the Pacific Northwest heat wave of 2021 coincided with 159 (95% detection interval = 122, 195) excess injury deaths in Washington State.

DISCUSSION

Our results show evidence of excess injury deaths after the 2021 Pacific Northwest heat wave, a 1-in-1000-years event caused by a ridge of high pressure resulting in a heat dome that trapped hot air over Washington State.[7] Anomalously warm temperatures plausibly influence injury deaths for several reasons. First, injury deaths vary seasonally in the United States,[11] which motivated us to explore whether temperature influences injury death rates. Second, plausible behavioral and physiological pathways exist

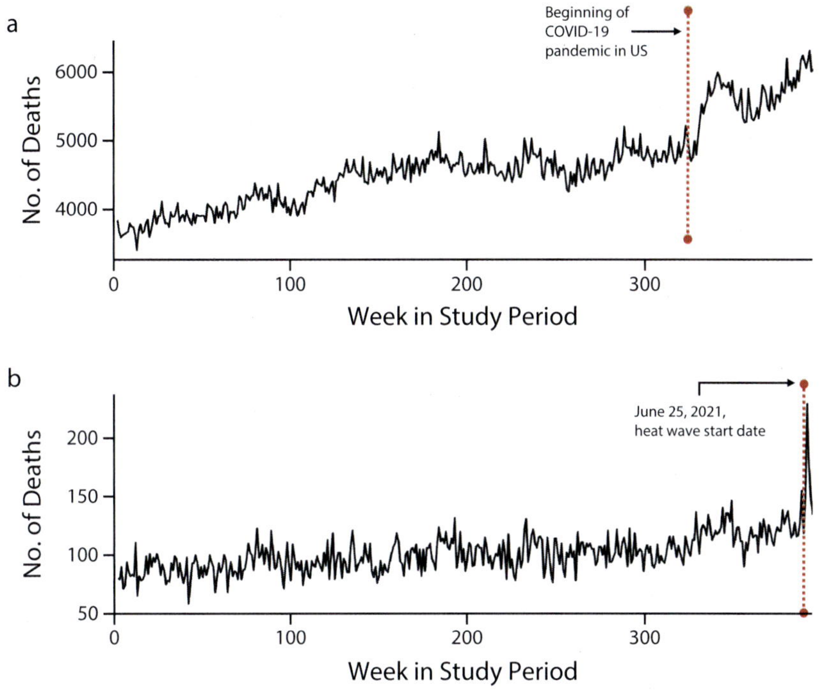

FIGURE 1— Observed Injury Deaths in (a) the United States and (b) Washington State: December 29, 2013–July 31, 2021

Note. The dashed red lines indicate the beginning of the COVID-19 pandemic (part a) and the beginning of the 2021 Pacific Northwest heat wave (part b). Observed injury deaths were obtained from the US Centers for Disease Control and Prevention and calculated as all-cause deaths minus "natural deaths."

for an association between temperature and injuries, such as changes in alcohol consumption, driving behavior, levels of anger and despair, and increased swimming.[12] Third, previous studies examining ambient temperature and injury outcomes in the United States have found positive associations.[2,3]

Public health programming during anomalously warm temperatures, intended to protect vulnerable communities from hazardous heat, should include ways to mitigate deaths from intentional injuries (such as assault and suicide) and unintentional injuries (such as falls, transport accidents, and drowning). Such programming will likely be needed more frequently given climate change.

We used provisional state-level death certificate data that do not specify cause or location of death (beyond state). Certain groups may be at disproportionate risk of the effects of heat, including older adults, workers, and others undertaking strenuous physical activity in uncooled spaces. Certain injury outcomes may also be more likely following heat exposure, but we could not disaggregate weekly injury deaths into subcategories (e.g., opioid-related mortality). Future studies should consider subcategories of injury and at-risk subgroups.

PUBLIC HEALTH IMPLICATIONS

Under climate scenarios with 2°C warming, models project that heat waves of this magnitude would occur every 5 to 10 years and that similar events would be 1.3°C hotter than today.[7] Public health interventions that broadly target the cause of injuries during periods of anomalously warm temperatures—for example, contacting isolated members of communities and campaigns promoting safe swimming or providing additional mental health services—should be a priority. *AJPH*

ABOUT THE AUTHORS

Joan A. Casey and Robbie M. Parks are with the Columbia University Mailman School of Public Health, New York, NY. Tim A. Bruckner is with the Program in Public Health, University of California, Irvine. Alison Gemmill is with the Johns Hopkins Bloomberg School of Public Health, Baltimore, MD. Ralph Catalano is with the School of Public Health, University of California, Berkeley.

CORRESPONDENCE

Correspondence should be sent to Joan A. Casey, PhD, MA, 3980 15th Ave NE, Room 254B, Seattle, WA 98105 (e-mail: jacasey@uw.edu). Reprints can be ordered at http://www.ajph.org by clicking the "Reprints" link.

PUBLICATION INFORMATION

Full Citation: Casey JA, Parks RM, Bruckner TA, Gemmill A, Catalano R. Excess injury mortality in Washington State during the 2021 heat wave. *Am J Public Health.* 2023;113(6):657–660.

Acceptance Date: February 19, 2023.

DOI: https://doi.org/10.2105/AJPH.2023.307269

CONTRIBUTORS

J. A. Casey and R. Catalano conceptualized the project. T. A. Bruckner and R. Catalano completed statistical analyses. J. A. Casey and R. M. Parks wrote the article. All authors provided feedback on analyses and article writing.

ACKNOWLEDGMENTS

This work was supported in part by the National Institutes of Environmental Health Sciences (R00ES027023, to J. A. Casey, and K99ES033742, to R. M. Parks).

CONFLICTS OF INTEREST

The authors have no conflicts of interest to report.

HUMAN PARTICIPANT PROTECTION

This research relied on publicly available data that were exempt from institutional review board review.

REFERENCES

1. Romanello M, McGushin A, Di Napoli C, et al. The 2021 report of the Lancet Countdown on health

and climate change: code red for a healthy future [erratum in *Lancet*. 2021;398(10317):2148]. *Lancet*. 2021;398(10311):1619–1662. https://doi.org/10.1016/S0140-6736(21)01787-6

2. Burke M, González F, Baylis P, et al. Higher temperatures increase suicide rates in the United States and Mexico. *Nat Clim Chang*. 2018;8(8): 723–729. https://doi.org/10.1038/s41558-018-0222-x
3. Parks RM, Bennett JE, Tamura-Wicks H, et al. Anomalously warm temperatures are associated with increased injury deaths. *Nat Med*. 2020; 26(1):65–70. https://doi.org/10.1038/s41591-019-0721-y
4. Lehmann F, Alary PE, Rey G, Slama R. Association of daily temperature with suicide mortality: a comparison with other causes of death and characterization of possible attenuation across 5 decades. *Am J Epidemiol*. 2022;191(12):2037–2050. https://doi.org/10.1093/aje/kwac150
5. Calkins MM, Bonauto D, Hajat A, et al. A case-crossover study of heat exposure and injury risk among outdoor construction workers in Washington State. *Scand J Work Environ Health*. 2019;45(6): 588–599. https://doi.org/10.5271/sjweh.3814
6. Spector JT, Bonauto DK, Sheppard L, et al. A case-crossover study of heat exposure and injury risk in outdoor agricultural workers. *PLoS One*. 2016;11(10):e0164498. https://doi.org/10.1371/journal.pone.0164498
7. Philip SY, Kew SF, Van Oldenborgh GJ, et al. Rapid attribution analysis of the extraordinary heat wave on the Pacific coast of the US and Canada in June 2021. *Earth Syst Dyn*. 2022;13(4):1689–1713. https://doi.org/10.5194/esd-13-1689-2022
8. US Energy Information Administration. Nearly 90% of US households used air conditioning in 2020. 2022. Available at: https://www.eia.gov/todayinenergy/detail.php?id=52558. Accessed January 4, 2023.
9. Weinberger KR, Harris D, Spangler KR, Zanobetti A, Wellenius GA. Estimating the number of excess deaths attributable to heat in 297 United States counties. *Environ Epidemiol*. 2020;4(3):e096. https://doi.org/10.1097/EE9.0000000000000096
10. US Centers for Disease Control and Prevention. Underlying cause of death, 1999–2018. Available at: https://wonder.cdc.gov/ucd-icd10.html. Accessed September 7, 2021.
11. Parks RM, Bennett JE, Foreman KJ, Toumi R, Ezzati M. National and regional seasonal dynamics of all-cause and cause-specific mortality in the USA from 1980 to 2016. *Elife*. 2018;7:e35500. https://doi.org/10.7554/eLife.35500
12. Gallop. Climate change and wellbeing around the world. 2022. Available at: https://www.gallup.com/analytics/397940/climate-change-and-wellbeing.aspx. Accessed August 31, 2022.

"Ashamed to Put My Name to It": Monsanto, Industrial Bio-Test Laboratories, and the Use of Fraudulent Science, 1969–1985

David Rosner, PhD, MSPH, and Gerald Markowitz, PhD

One of the most well-documented episodes of scientific manipulation and overt fraud was the scandal involving Industrial Bio-Test Laboratories (IBT) in the 1970s and the chronic toxicity tests it conducted on behalf of Monsanto that ultimately led to the indictment and conviction of employees of IBT and the Monsanto Corporation. IBT, at the time the nation's largest private laboratory, served a range of industries and government agencies. IBT conducted about 22 000 toxicology studies for scores of corporations, representing between 35% and 40% of all tests conducted in private labs in the country. IBT has been justly condemned for its fraudulent activities in the 1970s, but no one has looked at the relationship between the corporate funders of IBT's research and its fraudulent practices. We use previously secret corporate documents that detail the role of IBT's largest customer, Monsanto, which used fraudulent data to influence government. This material, revealed through legal discovery proceedings now under way regarding polychlorinated biphenyls (PCBs) and Roundup, show the long-lasting impact of Monsanto's behavior on efforts to regulate large corporations as well as on the long-term effects on human health. (*Am J Public Health*. 2023;113(6):661–666. https://doi.org/10.2105/AJPH.2023.307247)

AJPH June 2023, Vol 113, No. 6

For more than a century, organizations like the National Safety Council, the Industrial Health Foundation, and even the Manufacturing Chemists' Association representing the chemical industry, have pledged to test their products and guarantee the safety of materials introduced into the environment in exchange for limiting the reach of government regulators. If there were dangers, they promised to let users know what they were. Even after the establishment of the Occupational Safety and Health Administration (OSHA) and the Environmental Protection Agency (EPA) in 1970, the government largely depended on the integrity of industries to provide the necessary scientific data that could be used as the basis of relatively loose regulation.[1] This issue of the integrity of industry-sponsored science has become ever more important as discovery proceedings in court have released internal memos and studies revealing that industries—ranging from the tobacco, asbestos, and lead industries through the giant oil and chemical companies—have not been forthcoming about what they knew about the dangers of their products.[2] The creation of doubt in the science used to expose the danger, the hiding of information, and the misrepresentation of data to federal authorities have been the subject of numerous studies in recent years.[3]

One of the best-documented episodes of scientific manipulation and fraud was the scandal involving Industrial Bio-Test Laboratories (IBT), a private testing laboratory in Illinois, which in the early 1970s conducted long-term studies using rats on a variety of chemicals for various corporations, including Monsanto. In subsequent years, the uncovering of the corruption of these studies led to the indictment, conviction, and imprisonment of IBT and Monsanto employees.[4] In this article, we use previously secret corporate documents detailing the role of the

Monsanto Corporation, IBT's largest customer, in encouraging and engaging in fraudulent practices at IBT to thwart government investigations into the dangers of Monsanto's products on human health.[5]

In the late 1960s, Monsanto approached IBT to conduct chronic toxicity tests on polychlorinated biphenyls (PCBs) in response to growing national concern about the universal presence of PCBs in the environment. PCBs, a plasticizing and insulating agent widely used in paints, plastics, carbonless copy paper, adhesives, electrical transformers and capacitors, and numerous other products had been marketed by Monsanto for commercial use beginning in the 1930s. In the mid-1960s, it was identified in animal and human tissue, fish, waterways, and birds throughout the world, leading to demands for information as to its toxicity. Monsanto, which for nearly three decades had failed to test the long-term effects of PCBs on human health, turned to IBT to conduct chronic two-year toxicity testing on animals.[6] From the first, these studies were seen by Monsanto as part of a larger strategy to prove to the public and government—particularly the Food and Drug Administration (FDA) and the newly established EPA—that PCBs "do not constitute a serious threat to the public health" and specifically were not carcinogenic.[7]

Monsanto contracted with IBT in 1969 to perform two-year chronic toxicity studies and other studies, one of which did not meet the company's expectations as it did not turn out to be "as favorable as we [Monsanto] had hoped or anticipated. Particularly alarming is evidence of effect on hatchability and production of thin egg shells." Hence, Monsanto arranged with IBT to repeat "some of the studies" in order "to arrive at better conclusions."[8] They sent IBT new samples of their PCBs that they claimed were "clean[ed] up" and told IBT they hoped to "find a higher 'no effect' level," a potential "safe" level below which the experimental animals would not show symptoms of damage.[9] Indeed, their collaboration with IBT to downplay the hazards of PCBs appears to have been successful. By 1973, they claimed that "the most important data which has led the government agencies to permit the continued but constricted use of polychlorinated biphenyl are the extensive animal toxicity studies which we have completed in the last two years."[10]

FRAUDULENT LABORATORY PRACTICE

But the reliability of those studies was belied by two facts: first, the actual conditions in the IBT labs that tested PCBs for Monsanto were soon found to be compromised, and second, data were found to be fabricated and sent to the government as ostensible "proof" of their chemicals' safety.

Philip Smith, an assistant toxicologist in the IBT labs where PCB chronic toxicity studies were conducted, described the gross conditions under which the experimental animals were kept, which compromised the collection of reliable data: "[L]oose and wild [rats] . . . were in the rooms . . . chewing the feet off of the [experimental] animals that were in the cages." He explained it was "difficult to tell the difference between loose laboratory animals and loose [wild] animals that have been raised outside and gotten in," as interbreeding had occurred and technicians were not able to distinguish which rats were which. The poor professional standards maintained in the lab can be gleaned from Smith's description that "technicians . . . were caught burning rats' testicles with lit matches." Dead rats were often left to decompose so badly that they "would ooze through the bottom of their cages, and all their tissues would be at a total los[s] for any pathology work."[11] Animal caretakers reported "that there were many dead animals that were stinking so bad that [the] caretaker did not want to go into the room to change the water bottles" and new, live animals were substituted for dead ones with no acknowledgment.[12] Despite the obviously compromised test conditions, IBT produced seemingly scientifically rigorous reports on three of Monsanto's PCB products (Aroclor 1254, 1260, and 1242), claiming that testing proved PCBs were not carcinogenic.[13]

The second issue involved fraud: simply, IBT employees made up data. Otis Fancher, a toxicologist at IBT, wrote to his colleagues as early as 1972 that much of the work was so shoddy that he "was ashamed to publish the work done." He wrote that "much of the data are either fudged or collected with carelessness of incompetence, particularly the data for the supplementary studies of [PCBs]."[14] In fact, data reported were inaccurate or literally invented and the language was altered by Monsanto officials themselves. In 1975, IBT's Joseph C. Calandra sent a draft of their latest "AROCLOR 2-year Rat Feeding Studies" to George Levinskas, Monsanto's manager of environmental assessment and toxicology, listing Aroclor 1254 as being "slightly tumorigenic." Levinskas objected, asking that the phrasing be changed to "does not appear to be carcinogenic," a simple but important revision that avoided raising government concerns about cancer. Calandra complied.[15]

Central to these activities was Paul Wright, who was the link between IBT and Monsanto. Wright was employed at Monsanto beginning in 1965 as a senior research chemist and from 1968 until 1970 as a research group leader. In 1970, as IBT began its two-year chronic testing of PCBs for Monsanto, Wright moved to IBT, where he directed the toxicology lab that oversaw these studies. In late 1972, he returned to Monsanto as the toxicology manager and stayed at Monsanto until 1984, shortly before his conviction for having conspired to use the US Postal Service to defraud the government was upheld, and he was imprisoned.

Philip Smith, the lab assistant in the IBT PCB studies, gave vivid descriptions of how Wright had falsified data that ended up in the report sent to the government. "The body weight data [were] non-existent," Smith testified in one deposition he gave years later. "For intervals it was not collected."[16] He knew that, "because under Paul Wright's instruction, I plotted out the body weight data that we had in the department and all of the data that we could find in the storage area of the department. Then he [Wright] plotted out and gave me body weight numbers to put into the report for all the spaces that we had no records for." Smith "watched him" "make up numbers" "out of his head."[17] In 1976, the FDA found inconsistent data in one of IBT's studies, leading it to scrutinize IBT's studies.

In 1977, as questions about its studies accumulated, IBT requested a meeting with Monsanto about the chronic toxicity testing that they had conducted on several different substances. In July, Monsanto officials, including M. C. Throdahl, the company's group vice president for environmental policy and member of the Board of Directors, and Paul Wright, now having returned to Monsanto and soon to be director of its Environmental Health Laboratory, met with officials from IBT, including A. J. Frisque, its president, and F. R. Current, IBT's legal counsel. The "reason for the meeting," according to an internal Monsanto memo, was the "recent actions by the FDA and the EPA (pesticides) in questioning the validity of toxicology studies performed by IBT." The FDA had specifically questioned the studies performed on trichlorocarbanilide (TCC), an antibacterial agent that, based on IBT reports, the FDA had approved for use in soaps and lotions.[18] IBT reviewed its operations and "discovered . . . major problems . . . at IBT's Northbrook, Illinois, facility," where their long-term PCB and other chemical rodent studies were conducted.[19] At the meeting, Monsanto Vice President Throdahl "asked specifically whether 'fraud' was involved in the twelve" Monsanto long-term rodent studies, to which the president of IBT "replied that 'extrapolation' and 'faulty interpretations' were part of the problems . . . and that he guesses this constitutes 'fraud.'" Monsanto's representatives called this "a very damaging admission [that] was made in the presence of a [IBT] lawyer who took no exception to the question or answer."[20]

INDICTMENT AND CONVICTION

In the late 1970s and into the early 1980s, the US government investigated the toxicological work that had been done at IBT. On May 4, 1981, a federal grand jury handed down an indictment focused on TCC, one of the 12 Monsanto chemicals then being tested in the rat toxicology labs. The indictment charged former IBT president Joseph C. Calandra, Moreno L. Keplinger, Paul L. Wright (now back at Monsanto), and James B. Plank with fraud. The indictment charged that between 1970 and 1977, Wright and the others had

> devised and intended to devise a scheme to defraud clients and government agencies by writing and distributing false and fraudulent study reports and false and fraudulent explanations of study reports, and by concealing the fraudulent nature of the study reports and explanations of studies and study reports.[21]

The accusations focused on Wright, Keplinger, Plank, and Calandra, who had represented that the studies had lasted 24 months when in fact the defendants "knew that the report included data from a substantial number of animals that had been on the study for significantly lesser periods of time." The defendants were also accused of falsifying the report they sent to the federal government, creating inaccurate mortality tables "which the defendants then knew to be false in that it substantially under-reported . . . the number of animals that died during the study," and thus "concealed . . . that the animal mortality . . . was substantially greater than reported in any version of the study report."[22]

The indictment detailed that Monsanto's Wright made "false, fictitious and fraudulent statements and representations . . . and concealed and covered up material facts" on the "Two Year Chronic Oral Toxicity with TCC, trichlorocarbanilide." Wright, who by 1976 had returned to Monsanto as the company's "toxicology manager," falsely predated the study by two years, to March 21, 1974,[23] showing that he was aware of, and continued to engage in, fraud after he had returned to Monsanto.[24]

In January 1978, the FDA and the EPA investigated three other long-term studies that IBT had conducted, including two that were done for Monsanto on Machete, another Monsanto herbicide, and monosodium cyanurate (ACL). The FDA concluded that in both studies there was evidence that Monsanto knew of "significant problems" at IBT "prior to submitting their [Monsanto's] report to the US Government." There was "strong evidence of client's being knowledgeable of inaccuracies in the final report," and in the other IBT study of ACL there was "strong indication of client's knowledge of the deficiencies before they issued their report to the US Government." The inspectors reported that "anticipated toxicity problems known to both the client [Monsanto] and test facility [IBT] were deliberately overlooked."[25]

The trial of the four defendants began at the United States District Court in Chicago in April 1983 and continued for several months. Almost immediately, national and local newspapers picked up on the significance of the case, pointing out that it raised many questions about the integrity and honesty not only of IBT but of Monsanto itself. Monsanto's press office denied that Wright was guilty of any fraud: "We think Mr. Wright is innocent and if his case goes to trial, the trial will vindicate him."[26]

Monsanto's statements were disingenuous at best. As we have indicated, four years prior to the indictment in 1977, Monsanto had been bluntly told by IBT's president that studies Wright had directed at IBT were fraudulent. Nevertheless, in 1977 Monsanto promoted Wright to director of the Environmental Health Laboratory, and in 1981, when Wright was indicted, he was assigned to work on special projects, including overseeing its Material Safety Data Sheets, the documents that OSHA demanded be available to warn workers about dangers of substances they were handling.[27] Far from being reprimanded or fired, Wright was given merit raises in 1977, 1978, and 1980. In 1982, a year after he was indicted,[28] Monsanto paid his legal defense to the tune of $1.4 million.[29] Monsanto continued to cite these studies well into the future as evidence of the safety of PCBs. In 1979, for example, a Monsanto publication cited the IBT studies of PCBs as "the most comprehensive safety tests of the time."[30] Further, in 1983 and 1985 Monsanto continued to cite the IBT studies in their Material Safety Data Sheets.[31] As late as 2018, one of their experts in PCB litigation depended on these fraudulent studies.[32]

In August 1983, Paul Wright, Moreno L. Keplinger, and James B. Plank, former assistant toxicology manager, were convicted of fraud and sentenced to jail.[33] But even following conviction, Monsanto gave Wright a "golden parachute," providing him with full retirement benefits, accrued vacation time, one month's severance, and the services of a recruitment specialist to help him find future jobs when he was released from prison.[34]

CONCLUSION

In the period following the expansion of government regulation in the early 1970s, the government depended on the integrity of industries and their private laboratories to provide them with information needed to establish new standards. Hence, the EPA, OSHA, and the Consumer Product Safety Commission, along with older agencies like the FDA—government agencies with neither the resources nor the inclination to test the myriad chemicals and synthetic products yearly produced by US industry—depended on companies' integrity. Following the revelations discussed here, "Good Laboratory Practices Regulations" were promulgated that were intended to guarantee the quality of research upon which federal regulations depend.[35] But the central tension between the interests of industries and the interests of public health remained. Here, we show that the influence of industry on laboratory practices made the corruption of science more likely. With or without regulatory standards, we need to maintain vigilance over companies whose self-interest has distorted science and may continue to do so. AJPH

ABOUT THE AUTHORS

David Rosner is with the Department of Sociomedical Sciences, Mailman School of Public Health, and Department of History and the Center for the History & Ethics of Public Health, Columbia University, New York, NY. Gerald Markowitz is with the Department of Interdisciplinary Studies, John Jay College and the City University Graduate Center, New York.

CORRESPONDENCE

Correspondence should be sent to David Rosner, PhD, Ronald Lauterstein Professor, Center for the History & Ethics of Public Health, Mailman School of Public Health, 722 West 168th St Room 935, New York, NY 10032 (e-mail: dr289@cumc.columbia.edu). Reprints can be ordered at http://www.ajph.org by clicking the "Reprints" link.

PUBLICATION INFORMATION

Full Citation: Rosner D, Markowitz G. "Ashamed to put my name to it": Monsanto, Industrial Bio-Test Laboratories, and the use of fraudulent science, 1969–1985. *Am J Public Health*. 2023;113(6): 661–666.

Acceptance Date: January 22, 2023.

DOI: https://doi.org/10.2105/AJPH.2023.307247

CONTRIBUTORS

Both authors contributed equally to the research, writing, and conceptualization of the article.

ACKNOWLEDGMENTS

We thank our colleagues Merlin Chowkwanyun, Kavita Sivaramakrishnan, and Ronald Bayer for their thoughtful comments on our work.

CONFLICTS OF INTEREST

Both David Rosner and Gerald Markowitz have participated as expert witnesses in lawsuits on behalf of the City of Seattle, the State of Washington, and individuals regarding PCB cases against Monsanto

ENDNOTES

1. David Rosner and Gerald Markowitz, "'Educate the Individual . . . to a Sane Appreciation of the Risk': A History of Industry's Responsibility to Warn of Job Dangers Before the Occupational Safety and Health Administration," *American Journal of Public Health* 106 (January 2016): 28–35 (https://doi.org//10.2105/AJPH.2015.302912).
2. For examples of the types of historical internal documents made available through various court proceedings, see Columbia University's and CUNY's Web site http://www.toxicdocs.org, which provides millions of pages of internal corporate memos, private research studies, corporate statements and public relations materials, and more.
3. Robert Proctor, *The Golden Holocaust: Origins of Cigarette Catastrophe and the Case for Abolition* (Berkeley, CA: University of California Press, 2012); Allan Brandt, *The Cigarette Century: The Rise, Fall, and Deadly Persistence of the Product that Defined America* (New York, NY: Basic Books, 2009); Gerald Markowitz and David Rosner, *Deceit and Denial: the Deadly Politics of Industrial Pollution*, with a new epilogue (Berkeley, CA: University of California Press, 2013); Elena Conis, *How to Sell a Poison: The Rise, Fall, and Toxic Return of DDT* (New York, NY: Bold Type Books, 2022); Gerald Markowitz and David Rosner, *Lead Wars: The Politics of Science and the Fate of America's Children* (Berkeley, CA: University of California Press, 2010); David Michaels, *Doubt Is Their Product* (New York, NY: Oxford University Press, 2008); David Michaels, *The Triumph of Doubt: Dark Money and the Science of Deception* (New York, NY: Oxford University Press, 2020); Naomi Oreskes and Erik Conway, *Merchants of Doubt: How a Handful of Scientists Obscured the Truth on Issues From Tobacco Smoke to Global Warming* (New York, NY: Bloomsbury, 2010).
4. Eliot Marshall, "The Murky World of Toxicity Testing," *Science*, new series, 220 (June 10, 1983): 1130–1132 (https://doi.org/10.1126/science.6857237); Keith Schneider, "Faking It: The Case Against Industrial Bio-Test Laboratories," Natural Resources Defense Council, *Amicus Journal*, Spring 1983, republished in "Planet Waves," https://planetwaves.net/contents/faking_it.html; Edward Herman, "Corporate Sovereignty and (Junk) Science," *Z Magazine*, November 1998 (http://www.zcommunications.org/corporate-sovereignty-and-junk-science-by-edward-herman), accessed July 14, 2022; Editorial, "The Scandal in Chemical Testing," *New York Times*, May 16, 1983, Section A, p. 18 (https://www.nytimes.com/1983/05/16/opinion/the-scandal-in-chemical-testing.html), accessed January 3, 2023.
5. See *Michael Evard, Plaintiff, v Monsanto Company, et al., Defendants*, Circuit Court of Cook County, Illinois, Case No. 2019-L-011574; *Neal Frank v Monsanto Company, et al., Defendants*, First Judicial District Court, County of Santa Fe, State of New Mexico, No. D-101-cv-2021-00481. These cases involve polychlorinated biphenyls and Roundup, Monsanto's widely used pesticide. Keith Schneider, "Lab Fraud—or Government Harassment?", *Boston Globe*, April 3, 1983, p. A22; Keith Schneider, "Faking It, The Case Against Industrial Bio-Test Laboratories," in *The Amicus Brief* (Washington, DC: National Resources Defense Council, 1983). IBT, at the time the nation's largest private laboratory, was founded in 1953 by Joseph Calandra, a professor at Northwestern University, who organized three laboratories in the Chicago area to serve industry's need for testing new products. By the early 1970s it had conducted about 22 000 toxicology studies for scores of corporations, representing between 35% and 40% of all tests conducted in private labs in the country. "Nearly half of IBT's studies were used to support federal registrations of a mammoth array of products: insecticides, herbicides, food additives, chemicals for water treatment, cosmetics, pharmaceuticals, soaps and bleaches, even coloring for ice cream" (https://planetwaves.net/contents/faking_it.html), accessed January 4, 2023.
6. For a full discussion of the identification of PCBs as an environmental pollutant and Monsanto's response, see Gerald Markowitz and David Rosner, "Monsanto, PCBs, and the Creation of a 'World-Wide Ecological Problem,'" *Journal of Public Health Policy* 39 (2018): 463–540 (https://doi.org/10.1057/s41271-018-0146-8); for a detailed examination of Monsanto's history of PCB production and pollution, see Ellen Griffith Spears, *Baptized in PCBs: Race, Pollution, and Justice in an All-American Town* (Chapel Hill, NC: University of North Carolina Press, 2014).
7. "Report of the Aroclor 'Ad Hoc' Committee (Second Draft)," October 15, 1969, "Company Confidential Attorney-Client Privilege" (https://www.toxicdocs.org/d/QXGD7Vm44Jx8qdpk742948pp7?lightbox=1), accessed January 3, 2023; Markowitz and Rosner, "Monsanto, PCBs, and the Creation of a "World-Wide Ecological Problem.'"
8. "The PCB-Pollution Problem," January 21 and 22, 1970, meeting with General Electric Co. (https://cdn.toxicdocs.org/Ed/EdoyOJrmzBNJpQnGg36Oj3Y2j/EdoyOJrmzBNJpQnGg36Oj3Y2j.pdf), accessed January 3, 2023.
9. Wheeler to Otis Fancher, Director, IBT, May 25, 1970 (https://www.toxicdocs.org/d/YGBLJpeRa2jDEjL7MqLRzwZgn?lightbox=1), accessed January 3, 2023.
10. Wheeler to Wilbur H. Speicher, Administrator, Industrial Hygiene, Westinghouse, February 23, 1973 (https://www.toxicdocs.org/d/3Q77xYrYKbKJaL9XdERMR6zwx?lightbox=1), accessed January 3, 2023.
11. Deposition of Philip S. Smith, July 9, 1987, *Cecil Scott, et al., Plaintiffs, v Monsanto Company, Defendant*, in the United States District Court, Eastern District of Texas, Beaumont Division, B-84-1103-CA, p. 244, 253 (https://www.toxicdocs.org/d/1gvgbp82nx6rwMn1V4jZKrZYK?lightbox=1), accessed January 12, 2023.
12. Deposition of Philip S. Smith, July 9, 1987, *Cecil Scott, et al., Plaintiffs, v Monsanto Company, Defendant*, in the United States District Court, Eastern District of Texas, Beaumont Division, B-84-1103-CA, p. 254 (https://www.toxicdocs.org/d/1gvgbp82nx6rwMn1V4jZKrZYK?lightbox=1), accessed January 4, 2023.
13. Industrial Bio-Test, Laboratories, Inc., "Report to Monsanto Company, Two-Year Chronic Oral Toxicity With Aroclor 1254 in Albino Rats," Nov. 12, 1971, IBT No. B7298 (https://www.toxicdocs.org/d/2NNN6GKONbd0ezNzbge4O0bn7?lightbox=1), accessed February 14, 2023.
14. Otis Fancher to Don[avon] [Gordon], handwritten note, January 14, 1972, M 42627 (https://www.toxicdocs.org/d/ZJ55yDwBnqwJOq5QRqYxRoXdL?lightbox=1), accessed February 14, 2023.
15. George J. Levinskas to Joseph Calandra, "Re: Aroclor 2-Year Rat Feeding Studies," July 18, 1975 (https://www.toxicdocs.org/d/NNkDddqyXv6gR9LR4wJqn7oM8?lightbox=1), accessed January 10, 2023. J. C. Calandra to George Levinskas, "Re: Aroclor 2-Year Rat Studies," August 4, 1975 (https://www.toxicdocs.org/d/dQM4xXnvnXpg7rYaY46O7Lq96?lightbox=1), accessed January 10, 2023.
16. Deposition of Philip S. Smith, July 9, 1987, "Cecil Scott et al., Plaintiffs, vs. Monsanto Company, In the United States District Court Eastern District of Texas, Beaumont Division, B-84-1103-CA, MONSPCB0019134-19135, p. 183.
17. Deposition of Philip S. Smith, July 9, 1987, pp. 189–190. See also Trial Testimony of Philip Smith, October 28, 1991, WATER_PCB-00056547, pp. 1073–1074; see also ibid, pp. 1130–1137); United States District Court, Northern District of Illinois, Eastern Division, "United States v. Joseph Calandra, Moreno Keplinger, Paul Wright and James Plank," "Special October 1980 Grand Jury Charges," STLCOPCB80017757. See also Keith Schneider, "Faking It: The Case Against Industrial Bio-Test Laboratories," *The Amicus Journal*, Spring 1983, pp. 15–21 (https://www.toxicdocs.org/d/eybVeZMgomD8N3KRv1k41GJq?lightbox=1), accessed February 14, 2023.
18. W. Wayne Withers and G. Roush to M. C. Throdahl, July 13, 1977, PCB-ARCH075738 (https://www.toxicdocs.org/d/r3EnYLgeRGvQVrRwOQN7ev2q?lightbox=1), accessed January 6, 2023.
19. Ibid.
20. Ibid.
21. *The United States of America v Joseph C. Calandra, Moreno L. Keplinger, Paul L. Wright and James B. Plank*, Filed, May 4, 1981, United States District Court, Northern District of Illinois, Eastern Division, MONSPCB0021020-MONSPCB0021037 (https://www.toxicdocs.org/d/pp9be89q8qkoZEzzeR39R1V1d?lightbox=1), accessed February 14, 2023.
22. *The United States of America v. Joseph C. Calandra, Moreno L. Keplinger, Paul L. Wright and James B. Plank*, Filed, May 4, 1981, United States District Court, Northern District of Illinois, Eastern Division, May 4, 1981, MONSPCB0021025 (https://www.toxicdocs.org/d/pp9be89q8qkoZEzzeR39R1V1d?lightbox=1), accessed January 4, 2023.
23. Ibid.
24. Ibid.
25. FDA, EPA, Compliance Inspection, "Summary of Findings," January 16–March 9, 1978, MONSPCB0000621.
26. Keith Schneider, "Accused of Faking Data: Trial Set for Testing Firm, Monsanto Researcher," *St. Louis Post-Dispatch*, March 30, 1983, pp. 1, 10; see also Bill Richards, "Papers From Trial of Former IBT Officers Raise Many Questions on Product Safety," *Wall Street Journal*, May 13, 1983, pp. 31, 37; see also FDA, EPA, Compliance Inspection, "Summary of Findings," January 16–March 9, 1978, MONSPCB0000641.
27. January 1983 Performance Review and MONSPCB 0013836-39; Monsanto, Paul Wright "Employment History," MONSPCB0013764 (https://www.toxic

docs.org/d/2j2LykGJG84d0bJ4VkgGLanpL?lightbox=1), accessed July 14, 2022.

28. Monsanto, Paul Wright "Employment History."
29. Deposition of Richard W. Duesenberg, *Cecil Scott et al., Plaintiffs, v Monsanto Company*, In the United States District Court Eastern District of Texas, Beaumont Division, B-84-1103-CA. pp. 19-33, 47, MONSPCB002951-2965, 29279.
30. Monsanto Public Relations Department, Monsanto, Polychlorinated Biphenyls, PCBs, "A Report on Uses, Environmental and Health Effects and Disposal," Section 2, p. 4, [1979], WATER_PCB-SD0000063098 (https://www.toxicdocs.org/d/g242x7ZeNEwm0k5wRE8maLQRe?lightbox=1), accessed January 3, 2023.
31. Monsanto, Material Safety Data Sheet, "Polychlorinated Biphenyls," October 15, 1985, LEXOLDMON006373-63378; Monsanto Material Safety Data, September 15, 1980, MONS 000140; Monsanto Material Safety Data, October 15, 1985, MONS 003224 (https://www.toxicdocs.org/d/2qyQ8776EzvoG1d4R6Gz0EYpN?lightbox=1), accessed January 3, 2023.
32. See Oral and Video Deposition of John Schell, PhD., City of Hartford and Hartford Board of Education v. Monsanto Company, Solutia and Pharmacia, United States District Court, District of Columbia, January 11, 2018, pp. 27–43.
33. "Tighter Controls on Toxics Testing," *Chemical Week* 145 (August 24, 1983): 32–39.
34. *United States of America, Plaintiff-Appellee, v Moreno L. Keplinger, Paul Wright, and James B. Plank, Defendants-Appellants*, No. 84-1639, argued, April 25, 1985, decided, October 29, 1985. Following the conviction, Wright and the others appealed, and on October 29, 1985, the United States Court of Appeals upheld the convictions and noted that Wright committed some of the fraudulent acts while he was employed at Monsanto.
35. Good Laboratory Practice Regulations Management Briefings, Post Conference Report, August 1979, *Guidance for Industry*, August 1979 (https://www.fda.gov/regulatory-information/search-fda-guidance-documents/good-laboratory-practice-regulations-management-briefings-post-conference-report-aug-1979), accessed July 8, 2022.

Decreasing Survey Response Rates in the Time of COVID-19: Implications for Analyses of Population Health and Health Inequities

Nancy Krieger, PhD, Merrily LeBlanc, BA, Pamela D. Waterman, MPH, Sari L. Reisner, ScD, Christian Testa, BS, and Jarvis T. Chen, ScD

See also Kapadia, p. 618.

Objectives. To examine whether, and if so how, US national and state survey response rates changed after the onset of the COVID-19 pandemic.

Methods. We compared the change in response rates between 2020 and 2019 of 6 (3 social and economic, 3 health focused) major US national surveys (2 with state response rates).

Results. All the ongoing surveys except 1 reported relative decreases (~29%) in response rates. For example, the household response rate to the US Census American Community Survey decreased from 86.0% in 2019 to 71.2% in 2020, and the response rate of the US National Health Interview Survey decreased from 60.0% to 42.7% from the first to the second quarter of 2020. For all surveys, the greatest decreases in response rates occurred among persons with lower income and lower education.

Conclusions. Socially patterned decreases in response rates pose serious challenges and must be addressed explicitly in all studies relying on data obtained since the onset of the pandemic.

Public Health Implications. Artifactual reduction of estimates of the magnitude of health inequities attributable to differential response rates could adversely affect efforts to reduce these inequities. (*Am J Public Health*. 2023;113(6):667–670. https://doi.org/10.2105/AJPH.2023.307267)

AJPH June 2023, Vol 113, No. 6

Reckoning with the toll of the COVID-19 pandemic on population health requires addressing not only the direct harms caused—on both health and the societal determinants of health—but also the production of scientific knowledge about population health and health inequities.[1] In the United States, 1 issue concerns how survey response rates for surveys designed to be representative at the state or national level, as well as response rates for specific health investigations (e.g., on COVID-19 or other outcomes), have been affected by pandemic disruptions.[1–3] Also at issue are concurrent societal and institutional reckonings with structural racism precipitated by the police murder of George Floyd on May 25, 2020, combined with growing political and economic polarization, together affecting attitudes toward public health and other government agencies.[4–6]

A plausible scenario is that nonnegligible differential response rates[1,2] would be induced by the racialized and economic inequities in COVID-19's toll and the concomitant societal polarization.[1,7] Although at first not well documented, evidence now makes clear that, especially before vaccines became available and efforts to make them equitably accessible were funded and implemented, COVID-19 disproportionately infected people in low-wage jobs that required them to be physically present at work (typically with no sick leave) and, by extension, their family members.[2,7] Extant racialized economic occupational and residential segregation in turn led to disproportionately elevated COVID-19 rates in lower-income neighborhoods, especially those with higher concentrations of

Black, Latinx, and American Indian and Alaska Native residents, and among persons in institutional settings, including underresourced nursing homes and prisons.[2,7]

We accordingly examined whether, and if so how, response rates of major US national and state surveys changed after the onset of the COVID-19 pandemic. Three considerations motivated our inquiry: (1) the implications of any such impacts on response rates and the production of scientific knowledge about population health,[1,2] (2) the lack of any readily identifiable published articles documenting changes in response rates across numerous national surveys,[3] and (3) our awareness of the challenges our team faced in implementing a community-based study designed before COVID-19 for which recruitment began in March 2020, when the pandemic was declared a national emergency.[8]

METHODS

We focused on major US population data resources designed to be representative that are widely used in US population health and other population-based research. We included 6 national surveys conducted by the US Census, the US Department of Health and Human Services and agencies under its aegis (e.g., US National Center for Health Statistics, US Centers for Disease Control and Prevention), and the US Department of Labor, of which 2 provided data on response rates by states. The 6 surveys included are listed in Table 1 and their source information is provided in Table A (available as a supplement to the online version of this article at http://www.ajph.org).

We tallied the absolute and relative change in survey response rates, comparing data reported in the most recent prepandemic period (2019 to February 2020) to the data reported since the onset of the pandemic emergency period (after March 2020 to 2021, with 1 survey providing data for 2022). We also recorded the information provided, if any, about (1) changes in study design because of the pandemic, and (2) differential changes in response rates by social groups and discussion regarding weighting methodologies.

RESULTS

Among the 6 national surveys, 5 continued with reduced operation after March 2020, 1 halted operation entirely, and all but 1 reported notable reductions in response rates (Table 1). Comparing the 2020 with the 2019 data, the median absolute difference for the 9 national data points available was −15.6 percentage points (mean = −15.5%; range = −43.7 to −1.5), and the median relative change was 0.71 (mean = 0.77; range = 0.55–0.97); that is, a 29% lower response rate than in 2019. The survey least affected was the one that relied solely on remote interview methods before the pandemic (Behavioral Risk Factor Surveillance System; median absolute difference = −1.5%). The one with the greatest absolute decrease was the group quarters survey for the US Census American Community Survey (absolute difference = −47.2%). For the 4 surveys reporting 2021 response rates, the median relative difference was 0.91 and was smaller compared with 2019. For the 1 survey reporting data for 2022, the relative difference in response rates compared with 2019 was 0.87 (Table 1). Survey documentation consistently reported greater reductions in response rates among persons with lower income and lower educational attainment, as well as reduced coverage among Black and Hispanic populations. Three surveys (American Community Survey, Current Population Survey, and National Health Interview Survey) conducted analyses showing that standard weighting methods could not correct these problems (Table 1 and Table A).

DISCUSSION

In a context of societal disruptions owing to the COVID-19 pandemic, it is unsurprising that US national and state surveys have experienced substantial decreases in response rates, with 4 of the 5 major US surveys reporting relative reductions on the order of 29% (Table 1).[1–3] It is likewise not surprising that these reductions were socially patterned, with the greatest decreases among persons with lower income and lower education, and reduced coverage especially affecting the US Black and Hispanic populations (i.e., the social groups hardest hit by the onset of COVID-19; Table 1).[1–7]

Plausible hypotheses to explain these trends include (1) inabilities of survey staff to connect remotely with and enroll participants from whom data were previously obtained by in-person interviews, including persons in households without telephones and persons residing in group quarters (Table 1); and (2) increased respondent burden and distrust linked to the heightened weariness and wariness among persons whose lives and livelihoods were adversely affected by the pandemic[1,2,4,7,9] combined with heightened polarization about government agencies and their work.[5,6] Preliminary data suggest similar problems have affected project-specific health investigations that enrolled participants during the pandemic.[2,9]

TABLE 1— Response Rates Immediately Before and During the COVID-19 Pandemic for US National and State Social and Health Surveys Designed to Be Representative of the Population: 2019–2022

	Response Rates, %			Absolute Difference in Response Rates, Percentage Points		Relative Difference in Response Rates vs 2019	
	Immediately Prepandemic	Pandemic Time 1 (2020)	Pandemic Time 2 (2021)	Time 1 vs Prepandemic	Time 2 vs Prepandemic	Time 1 vs Prepandemic	Time 2 vs Prepandemic
US Census ACS (http://bit.ly/3ZDfyMM)[a]							
US housing units	86.0	71.2	85.3	−14.8	−0.7	0.83	0.91
US group quarters[b]	90.9	47.2	74.8	−43.7	−16.1	0.52	0.82
State housing units[c]							
Median	87.0	73.0	87.1	−14.0	0.10	0.83	1.00
Minimum	75.4	63.1	75.9	−12.3	0.10	0.84	1.00
Maximum	92.0	85.2	92.7	−6.8	0.70	0.93	1.00
State group quarters[b,c]							
Median	93.0	50.4	80.2	−36.6	−12.8	0.54	0.86
Minimum	65.3	28.9	35.5	−36.4	−29.8	0.49	0.54
Maximum	98.2	70.9	95.7	−27.3	−2.5	0.72	0.97
US Current Population Survey (http://bit.ly/3FcDXAJ)[a]							
United States	82.3	76.2	72.0	−6.1	−10.3	0.93	0.87
US Bureau of Labor Statistics: Consumer Expenditure Surveys (http://bit.ly/3YBOPz1)[a]							
Diary	49.5	33.9	NA	−15.6	NA	0.68	NA
Interview	52.2	45.8	NA	−6.4	NA	0.88	NA
US National Health Interview Survey (https://bit.ly/3J7gstZ)[a]							
Household	60.0	42.7	NA	−17.3	NA	0.71	NA
Adult sample	57.9	41.1	NA	−16.8	NA	0.71	NA
Child sample	57.6	40.1	NA	−17.5	NA	0.70	NA
US National Health and Nutrition Examination Survey (http://bit.ly/3Yz6LtY)[a]							
Screener response	85.3	NA	NA	NA	NA	NA	NA
Interview	49.6	NA	NA	NA	NA	NA	NA
Examination	44.0	NA	NA	NA	NA	NA	NA
BRFSS Survey (2019: https://bit.ly/40ijd2v; 2020: https://bit.ly/3LAxUK8; 2021: https://bit.ly/3Z2Ncur)							
United States							
Mean	50.0	47.8	44.6	−2.2	−5.4	0.96	0.89
Median	49.4	47.9	44.0	−1.5	−5.4	0.97	0.89
Minimum	37.3	34.5	23.5	−2.8	−13.8	0.92	0.63
Maximum	73.1	67.2	60.5	−5.9	−12.6	0.92	0.83

Note. ACS = American Community Survey; BRFSS = Behavioral Risk Factor Surveillance System; NA = not available. Relative times (immediately prepandemic, pandemic time 1, and pandemic time 2) vary by survey. See Table A (available as a supplement to the online version of this article at https://www.ajph.org) for full dates.

[a]Concerns stated in the survey documentation regarding social differentials in response rates, including inability to correct for these differentials using conventional weighting approaches (see Table A for descriptions). Each of these surveys additionally reported changes in survey design in response to the COVID-19 pandemic (see Table A for descriptions).

[b]Defined by the ACS report as "places where people live or stay in a group living arrangement that is owned or managed by an organization providing housing and/or services for the residents . . . such as college residence halls, residential treatment centers, skilled nursing facilities, group homes, military barracks, prisons, and worker dormitories" (http://bit.ly/3ZDfyMM).

[c]For the state-level ACS response rates, states include 50 US states plus the District of Colombia and Puerto Rico.

Socially patterned differential decreases in survey response rates threaten capacity for accurate investigation of trends in and analysis of population health, health inequities, and societal determinants of health.[1–3,9–11] Of concern is the potential impact on the range of values observed, the associations between the variables that predict selection and other variables of interest, and the population data need for reweighting,[11] with 3 surveys documenting the inability of conventional weighting methods to correct these problems (Table 1 and Table A).

One additional concern warranting investigation is how differentially decreasing response rates could lead to artifactual reduction of estimates of the magnitude of health inequities (e.g., if persons most harmed by societal injustice disproportionately are absent from the data or, if enrolled, have missing data not at random).[1,9,10] Such scenarios are plausible, given concerns about data quality documented in Table 1 and could undercut efforts to reduce these inequities. Rectifying the impacts of structural racism and other types of injustice on population health monitoring and the scientific production of public health and biomedical knowledge entails addressing these challenges.[1,4,7,10,12]

In summary, the COVID-19 pandemic has magnified existing challenges of recruitment, enrollment, and data analysis and has presented new challenges for public health agencies and researchers.[2,3,9–11] It is incumbent on those who undertake population surveys and those who undertake health research to explicitly situate the societal context, including the pandemic and sociopolitical context, in which participants provided data, the impacts on response rates and missing data, and implications for analyzing population health data and health inequities. AJPH

ABOUT THE AUTHORS

Nancy Krieger, Pamela D. Waterman, Sari L. Reisner, Christian Testa and Jarvis T. Chen are with the Harvard T.H. Chan School of Public Health, Boston, MA. Merrily LeBlanc is with Fenway Health, Boston, MA.

CORRESPONDENCE

Correspondence should be sent to Nancy Krieger, PhD, Professor of Social Epidemiology, American Cancer Society Clinical Research Professor, Department of Social and Behavioral Sciences, Harvard T.H. Chan School of Public Health, Kresge 717, 677 Huntington Ave, Boston, MA 02115 (e-mail: nkrieger@hsph.harvard.edu). Reprints can be ordered at http://www.ajph.org by clicking the "Reprints" link.

PUBLICATION INFORMATION

Full Citation: Krieger N, LeBlanc M, Waterman PD, Reisner SL, Testa C, Chen JT. Decreasing survey response rates in the time of COVID-19: implications for analyses of population health and health inequities. *Am J Public Health*. 2023;113(6): 667–670.

Acceptance Date: February 19, 2023.

DOI: https://doi.org/10.2105/AJPH.2023.307267

CONTRIBUTORS

N. Krieger led conceptualization and data collection and wrote the first draft of the article. M. LeBlanc assisted with data collection. M. LeBlanc, P. D. Waterman, S. L. Reisner, C. Testa, and J. T. Chen participated in discussions regarding article content and provided critical input into revising the draft text. All authors approve the final version for submission.

ACKNOWLEDGMENTS

This work was supported by the National Institutes of Health (grant 1R01MD012793; to N. K.).

CONFLICTS OF INTEREST

None of the authors has any conflicts of interest to declare.

HUMAN PARTICIPANT PROTECTION

No protocol approval was necessary because this brief report involved no human participants.

REFERENCES

1. Krieger N. Counting for accountability in a time of catastrophe: COVID-19 and other deaths, cohorts, color lines, and dollar signs. *Am J Public Health*. 2021;111(suppl 2):S91–S92. https://doi.org/10.2105/AJPH.2021.306257
2. Kennedy EB, Charifson M, Jehn M, Jensen EA, Vikse J. Prospective sampling bias in COVID-19 recruitment methods: experimental evidence from a national randomized survey testing recruitment materials. *BMC Med Res Methodol*. 2022;22(1):251. https://doi.org/10.1186/s12874-022-01726-2
3. Williams D. Survey nonresponse: trends, challenges, and strategies. December 9, 2022. Available at: https://apps.bea.gov/fesac/meetings/2022-12-09/Williams-Survey%20Response.pdf. Accessed December 11, 2022.
4. Krieger N. ENOUGH: COVID-19, structural racism, police brutality, plutocracy, climate change—and time for health justice, democratic governance, and an equitable sustainable future. *Am J Public Health*. 2020;110(11):1620–1623. https://doi.org/10.2105/AJPH.2020.305886
5. Ternullo S. "I'm not sure what to believe": media distrust and opinion formation during the COVID-19 pandemic. *Am Polit Sci Rev*. 2022;116(3):1096–1109. https://doi.org/10.1017/S000305542200003X
6. Hegland A, Zhang AL, Zichettella B, Pasek P. A partisan pandemic: how COVID-19 was primed for polarization. *Ann Am Acad Pol Soc Sci*. 2022; 700(1):55–72. https://doi.org/10.1177/00027162221083686
7. US Department of Health and Human Services. Presidential COVID-19 Health Equity Task Force: final report and recommendations. October 2021. Available at: https://www.minorityhealth.hhs.gov/assets/pdf/HETF_Report_508_102821_9am_508Team%20WIP11-compressed.pdf. Accessed February 7, 2023.
8. Krieger N. Advancing novel methods to measure and analyze multiple types of discrimination for population health research. Available at: https://reporter.nih.gov/search/T1qnoiJCukWRK0Mcvk-CJA/project-details/10330589. Accessed February 7, 2023.
9. Hathaway CA, Chavez MN, Kadono M, et al. Improving electronic survey response rates among cancer center patients during the COVID-19 pandemic: mixed methods pilot study. *JMIR Cancer*. 2021;7(3):e30265. https://doi.org/10.2196/30265
10. King C, Englander H, Priest KC, Korthuis PT, McPherson S. Addressing missing data in substance use research: a review and data justice-based approach. *J Addict Med*. 2020;14(6): 454–456. https://doi.org/10.1097/ADM.0000000000000644
11. Smith LH. Selection mechanisms and their consequences: understanding and addressing selection bias. *Curr Epidemiol Rep*. 2020;7(4):179–189. https://doi.org/10.1007/s40471-020-00241-6
12. National Institutes of Health. Ending structural racism: UNITE. October 20, 2022. Available at: https://www.nih.gov/ending-structural-racism/unite. Accessed February 7, 2023.

Substance Use Among Asian American Adults in 2016–2020: A Difference-in-Difference Analysis of a National Survey on Drug Use and Health Data

Yueqi Yan, PhD, Mieko Yoshihama, PhD, Jun Sung Hong, PhD, and Fan Jia, PhD

See also Wu, p. 604.

Objectives. To compare substance use among Asian American adults in 2020, when anti-Asian violence increased, with substance use among the same group during the previous 4 years and compare this with that of non-Hispanic Whites.

Methods. Using data from the National Survey on Drug Use and Health, 2016 to 2020, we investigated changes in substance use among Asian Americans compared with non-Hispanic Whites before and during the COVID-19 pandemic. We performed difference-in-difference analyses to estimate adjusted changes in past-month substance use in the 2 groups.

Results. The incidence rate ratio (IRR) among Asian Americans' past-month alcohol use, cocaine use, and tranquilizer misuse in 2020 versus in 2016 to 2019 was 1.3 times, 3.0 times, and 17.2 times, respectively, the same IRR among Whites.

Conclusions. The significant increase in misuse of several substances among Asian Americans relative to Whites in 2020 calls for careful assessment, identification, and treatment of this understudied population group.

Public Health Implications. Besides increasing Asian substance users' access to socioculturally responsive treatment programs, policy and resources should be focused on multilevel violence prevention efforts such as antiracial discrimination public education programs. (*Am J Public Health.* 2023;113(6):671–679. https://doi.org/10.2105/AJPH.2023.307256)

AJPH June 2023, Vol 113, No. 6

Racial discrimination against Asian Americans has a long history in the United States. Since the beginning of the COVID-19 pandemic, however, anti-Asian harassment and discrimination incidents have drastically increased. In 2020, some political leaders blamed specific Asian ethnic groups for "spreading the virus" by repeatedly using phrases such as "the Chinese virus" and "the Wuhan virus."[1,2] According to the latest report by Stop AAPI Hate, a US-based national organization, from March 2020 to March 2022, the organization received 11 467 reports of anti-Asian discrimination incidents.[3] Recent data from a nationally representative survey showed that 1 in 5 Asian Americans experienced a hate incident (e.g., verbal harassment, shunning, physical assault) in 2020 or 2021.[4]

Although direct exposure to racial/ethnic harassment and discrimination incidents has a wide range of health consequences,[5] secondary exposure (e.g., having family and friends who have been victimized) can also negatively affect individuals' mental health.[6] During the pandemic, media coverage of such incidents grew nationwide. Previous politically sanctioned hatred also reinforced racist and xenophobic public sentiments, positioning Asians as the "hated other."[7] All Asian American groups have potentially been exposed to elevated levels of toxic environmental stress, regardless of where they live and whether they have personally experienced such an incident. This could result in fear, depression, anxiety, or traumatic stress, which may trigger substance use to cope with these feelings.[8] Although the association of direct experience with racial discrimination and substance use has been well documented in the research literature,[6,9,10] relatively few studies have examined the effect on substance use of indirect exposure to racial discrimination via various media channels. One strategy for doing so is to compare the population estimate of the incidence and prevalence of substance use among Asian Americans before and during the pandemic, when anti-Asian hate incidents increased dramatically.

Although Asian Americans have historically reported lower rates of substance use, especially illicit drug use, than have Whites and other racial groups, several studies have demonstrated a compelling link between perceived race-based discrimination and substance use among minority groups.[11–13] Based on the tension-reduction model,[14] stress-coping theories,[15] and general strain theory,[16] substance use can function as a coping strategy for reducing stress associated with racial discrimination among minority groups. Previous studies also documented a higher risk of smoking among African American young adults,[17] alcohol use among US-born Latinos and African Americans,[18] and prescription drug misuse and lifetime marijuana and cocaine use among African American adults[18–20] when experiencing discrimination. A few studies have examined the relationship between racial discrimination and substance use among Asian Americans. Yoo et al.[17] found that Asian Americans treated as outsiders because of their race were at an increased risk of tobacco use.[21] Racial discrimination against Filipino Americans was positively associated with illicit drug use.[22] Recent studies further revealed that when experiencing discrimination, Asian Americans reported the highest misuse of pain relievers, tranquilizers, and stimulants among all minority groups.[20,23]

Data on substance use or misuse among Asian Americans during the pandemic are minimal, even though the pandemic began in 2020 and Asian Americans have been vulnerable to hate crimes and racial/ethnic discrimination. We compared changes in substance use or misuse among a nationally representative sample of Asian American adults in 2020 with their substance use or misuse in the previous 4 years. We hypothesized that Asian American adults experienced a higher rate of increase in substance use or misuse in 2020 compared with their substance use in the previous 4 years than did White Americans.

METHODS

In this retrospective cohort study, we used cross-sectional data from the National Survey on Drug Use and Health (NSDUH) from 2016 to 2020. The NSDUH is an annual population-based survey conducted in all 50 states and the District of Columbia that focuses on estimating the use of tobacco, alcohol, prescription psychotherapeutic, and other drugs by the US noninstitutionalized population aged 12 years and older. More methodological details are presented in the NSDUH *Methodological Summary and Definitions* report.[24]

We selected a sample of adults aged 18 years and older who self-identified as non-Hispanic Asian American or non-Hispanic White. We excluded individuals of more than 1 race/ethnicity from the study. We combined annual NSDUH data sets from 2016 to 2020, resulting in a total of 130 814 adults, including 42 625, 42 554, 43 026, 42 739, and 27 170 individual responses from 2016 to 2020, respectively. Because of the lockdown during the second and third quarters of the pandemic, data in 2020 were primarily collected in quarters 1 and 4, resulting in a smaller sample size than that of the 2016 to 2019 data, when data were collected in all 4 quarters. A majority of respondents were non-Hispanic White adults (n = 120 087, or 92%). The rest comprised 10 727 non-Hispanic Asian American adults (n = 10 727, or 8%).

Measures

Outcome measures included a series of survey responses related to self-reported, past-month use or misuse of substances, which was previously reported to be associated with racial discrimination–related, stress-coping behaviors.[16–20,22,23] They included the use or misuse of cigarettes, alcohol, marijuana, cocaine, methamphetamines, pain relievers, tranquilizers, stimulants, and sedatives as well as engaging in binge drinking. We defined binge drinking as drinking 5 or more drinks on the same occasion for everyone, regardless of gender. We assessed outcome measures of each type of substance by (1) number of days of engaging in a given behavior, with responses ranging from 0 to 30 days[24]; and (2) whether an individual was engaged in a given behavior or not (yes or no). We dummy-coded the racial groups as Asian Americans (1) and non-Hispanic White Americans (0). We created a dichotomous time measure to denote the 4 years before the COVID-19 pandemic (2016–2019; 0) and the year during the pandemic (2020; 1).

For control variables, we included sociodemographic and clinical confounding characteristics associated with substance use based on previous studies; we also matched Asian American and non-Hispanic White samples on these variables. We categorized individuals' age into 5 groups: 18 to 25 years, 26 to 34 years, 35 to 49 years, 50 to 64 years, and 65 years and older. We expressed a 4-level education variable as less than high school, high school graduation, some college, and college graduation or above. We categorized employment status as full-time, part-time, no work, and other work. We categorized total family household income into 4 groups: less than \$20 000, \$20 000 to \$49 999, \$50 000 to \$74 999, and \$75 000 or more. We recorded marital status in 4 groups: single, married, divorced, and widowed. We coded place of residence as large metro area, small metro area, or nonmetro area. We also included a binary measure of having health insurance coverage (1) or not (0) and a self-rated overall health measure on a 4-point scale ranging from excellent (1) to fair or poor (4).

Analytic Techniques

To examine how the incidents of substance use in 2020 differed from those of previous years for Asian Americans compared with White Americans, we generated propensity score (PS) weighting and then performed difference-in-difference (DID) analyses. To control for the time difference or effect, we first conducted separate logistic regression models to calculate year-specific PSs for Asian Americans versus White Americans. We weighted the PS models using survey sampling weights and strata so that the PSs were nationally representative.[25]

We further generated PS-adjusted sampling weights based on the product of the weighted odds of being Asian American versus White multiplied by the NSDUH survey sampling weights. The new weights balanced Asian Americans and White Americans on all the sociodemographic and clinical characteristics. This approach involves sampling weights in propensity score and outcome estimation stages and results in a PS-adjusted estimator that is resilient to various conditions that lead to selection bias.[26] The mean, SD, and ranges were 16436.09, 18581.50, and (5.0, 223960.30) for survey sampling weights and 10100.70, 18574.20, and (0.2, 217592.00) for PS-adjusted weights, respectively. We evaluated the post hoc balance estimation between Asian Americans and White Americans via the standardized difference in mean values for each covariate before and after PS weighting.[27]

Next, we calculated the changes in nationwide estimates of past-month substance use or misuse among Asian Americans versus non-Hispanic White Americans by comparing the frequency of past-month use of each substance in 2016 to 2019 versus in 2020. Given excessive counts of no self-reported past-month drug use, we performed zero-inflated Poisson regression and logistic regression analyses. Our aim was to conduct DID analyses, and estimate adjusted changes in past-month drug use and adjusted odds of past-month drug use, respectively. In the zero-inflated Poisson models, the incidence rate ratio (IRR) of the difference (2016–2019 vs 2020) in difference (Asian vs White Americans) represents the adjusted change rate of the risk of using or misusing each substance among Asian Americans relative to that of non-Hispanic White Americans before versus during the pandemic. We used the PS-adjusted weights in all the DID models to generate nationally representative estimates for each type of substance use.[24]

We also controlled sociodemographic and clinical characteristics to obtain doubly robust estimates of the change in past-month substance use or misuse among Asian Americans compared with non-Hispanic White Americans and predicted the excess zeros. Double robust estimates for a DID analysis incorporate both PS and outcome estimation and examine the actual average difference in outcome change rate over time between the 2 racial groups, even if either the PS model or the outcome model is misspecified.[28] We conducted sensitivity analyses using imputed and original substance use data to ensure that the significant change was not driven by imputation. The NSDUH *Methodological Summary and Definitions* report provide details about the imputation approach.[24]

RESULTS

Table 1 presents the sample characteristics of Asian and White American adults. Before PS weighting, both racial groups were significantly different on all the control variables except for gender and health insurance coverage. However, after we used the PS-adjusted weights, all the control variables were not significantly different between the 2 groups; this is evidence of well-balanced samples in both groups. Table 2 and Figures A and B (available as a supplement to the online version of this article at http://www.ajph.org) present the average frequency of past-month substance use or misuse and the percentage of any use or misuse for Asian American and White American adults from 2016 to 2020 after applying the

TABLE 1— Sample Characteristics of Asian American and Non-Hispanic White Adults: National Survey on Drug Use and Health, United States, 2016–2020

Variable	Non-Hispanic Asian (n = 10 727), %	Non-Hispanic White (n = 120 087)			
		Unweighted, %[a]	P	Weighted, %[b]	P
Gender			.17		.73
Female	52.6	51.4		52.9	
Male	47.4	48.6		47.1	
Age group, y			< .001		.99
18–25	15.1	11.6		15.3	
26–34	20.1	14.1		20.0	
35–49	30.6	22.6		30.4	
50–64	20.0	26.9		20.1	
≥ 65	14.2	24.9		14.2	
Education			< .001		> .99
< high school	6.7	7.7		6.8	
High school graduation	12.5	24.7		12.4	
Some college	21.1	31.8		21.1	
College graduation	59.7	35.8		59.7	
Employment			< .001		.88
Full-time	52.5	48.9		52.7	
Part-time	13.7	13.3		13.6	
No work	4.2	3.0		3.9	
Other work	29.6	34.7		29.8	
Total family income, $			< .001		> .99
< 20 000	11.5	12.1		11.4	
20 000–49 999	21.0	26.3		21.0	
50 000–74 999	13.2	16.4		13.1	
≥ 75 000	54.4	45.2		54.5	
Marital status			< .001		> .99
Single	28.1	23.8		28.3	
Married	62.7	55.4		62.5	
Divorced	3.1	6.6		6.2	
Widowed	6.2	14.2		3.0	
Living area			< .001		.91
Large metro	80.1	48.6		80.3	
Small metro	17.6	33.1		17.4	
Nonmetro	2.3	18.3		2.2	
Health insurance coverage			0.06		.96
Yes	94.1	93.3		94.1	
No	5.9	6.7		5.9	
Overall health condition			< .001		> .99
Excellent	26.8	20.5		27.0	
Very good	38.8	38.6		38.8	
Good	26.7	28.1		26.4	
Fair or poor	7.7	12.8		7.8	

Note. Sample size was n = 130 814.

[a]Unweighted refers only to propensity score weighting. Percentages were survey-weighted to be nationally representative and may not add up to 100.
[b]Weighted refers to propensity score–adjusted weighting. Percentages were weighted using the propensity score–adjusted weights.

TABLE 2— Past-Month Substance Use or Misuse Before and During the Pandemic Among Asian vs White Americans: National Survey on Drug Use and Health, United States, 2016–2020

Substance	Non-Hispanic White 2016 Mean[a] (SE)	2016 %[b]	2017 Mean[a] (SE)	2017 %[b]	2018 Mean[a] (SE)	2018 %[b]	2019 Mean[a] (SE)	2019 %[b]	2020 Mean[a] (SE)	2020 %[b]	Asian American 2016 Mean[a] (SE)	2016 %[b]	2017 Mean[a] (SE)	2017 %[b]	2018 Mean[a] (SE)	2018 %[b]	2019 Mean[a] (SE)	2019 %[b]	2020 Mean[a] (SE)	2020 %[b]
Cigarettes	3.79 (0.11)	17.9	3.40 (0.10)	16.5	3.44 (0.10)	16.4	3.23 (0.10)	15.4	3.61 (0.24)	15.3	1.73 (0.18)	9.4	1.59 (0.18)	8.5	1.43 (0.23)	8.7	1.37 (0.20)	8.1	1.91 (0.48)	12.5
Alcohol	6.43 (0.13)	68.8	6.33 (0.69)	68.5	6.22 (0.67)	67.7	6.16 (0.11)	66.9	5.65 (0.41)	62.9	1.92 (0.41)	38.0	2.55 (0.19)	41.4	2.89 (0.31)	43.3	2.42 (0.16)	40.9	2.93 (0.42)	36.9
Binge drinking	1.36 (0.04)	32.2	1.32 (0.04)	31.5	1.34 (0.04)	31.2	1.23 (0.05)	30.3	1.24 (0.05)	25.6	0.40 (0.05)	13.9	0.37 (0.04)	13.9	0.44 (0.04)	15.4	0.44 (0.05)	14.8	0.49 (0.07)	13.4
Marijuana	1.47 (0.07)	10.6	1.55 (0.06)	11.2	1.79 (0.07)	12.6	1.88 (0.07)	13.5	2.10 (0.10)	13.6	0.42 (0.06)	3.4	0.35 (0.06)	3.8	0.06 (0.13)	6.1	0.45 (0.06)	4.5	0.61 (0.15)	4.3
Cocaine	0.04 (0.01)	1.1	0.04 (0.01)	1.0	0.05 (0.01)	1.1	0.04 (0.01)	0.9	0.03 (0.01)	0.8	0.01 (0.00)	0.4	0.01 (0.01)	0.4	0.02 (0.01)	0.6	0.02 (0.01)	0.5	0.03 (0.03)	0.2
Pain reliever misuse	0.11 (0.01)	1.5	0.10 (0.01)	1.3	0.08 (0.01)	1.1	0.08 (0.01)	1.1	0.07 (0.01)	0.9	0.01 (0.01)	0.1	0.04 (0.01)	0.4	0.01 (0.00)	0.3	0.01 (0.01)	0.4	0.03 (0.03)	0.4
Tranquilizer misuse	0.05 (0.01)	1.2	0.05 (0.01)	1.0	0.04 (0.01)	0.8	0.05 (0.01)	1.0	0.03 (0.01)	0.8	0.002 (0.00)	0.1	0.002 (0.00)	<0.001	0.001 (0.00)	<0.001	0.002 (0.01)	<0.001	0.09 (0.09)	0.3
Stimulant misuse	0.06 (0.01)	1.3	0.07 (0.01)	1.3	0.05 (0.01)	1.0	0.06 (0.01)	1.1	0.06 (0.01)	1.1	0.002 (0.00)	0.2	0.01	0.3	0.03 (0.01)	0.8	0.01 (0.01)	0.3	0.04 (0.03)	0.3

Note. Sample size was n = 130 814. Frequency of sedative misuse was too low to estimate and therefore was not included.

[a]Mean and SE of the number of days using or misusing substances in the past month were estimated using combined propensity score weight with sampling weight data.

[b]Percentage of individuals using or misusing substances in the past month was estimated using combined propensity score weight with sampling weight data.

PS-adjusted weights. The reported average frequency of all substance use or misuse among Asian Americans was lower than that of White Americans. However, except for marijuana use, the use of most substances by White Americans did not increase linearly.

Before 2020, White Americans decreased cigarette and alcohol use and pain reliever misuse but increased marijuana use. Use of the other substances either increased and then decreased or the opposite. By contrast, Asian Americans' use or misuse of most substances decreased and then increased before 2020, except that cigarette use decreased and cocaine use increased consistently. Notably, Asian Americans' use or misuse of most substances increased considerably in 2020—especially compared with data from 2018 and 2019—except for marijuana use and pain reliever misuse.

Figure 1 presents adjusted estimates comparing Asian Americans' past-month substance use with that of White Americans based on the results of DID analyses using zero-inflated Poisson regression and logistic regression models. After we used the PS-adjusted weights and controlled for covariates, the ratio of the IRR of alcohol use for 2020 versus 2016 to 2019 among Asian Americans to the same IRR among White Americans was 1.3 (95% confidence interval [CI] = 1.1, 1.7). The ratio of IRR of cocaine use over time among Asian Americans to the same IRR among White Americans was 3.0 (95% CI = 1.2, 7.5). The IRR of tranquilizer use not directed by a medical doctor among Asian Americans over time was 17.2 times (95% CI = 5.4, 55.0) the same IRR among White Americans. However, there were no differences between Asian Americans and non-Hispanic White Americans in the IRR of cigarette a

Past-Month Use		IRR (95% CI)
Cigarettes	Imputed	1.0 (0.9, 1.2)
	Unimputed	1.0 (0.9, 1.0)
Alcohol	Imputed	1.3 (1.1, 1.7)
	Unimputed	1.3 (1.1, 1.7)
Binge drinking	Imputed	1.2 (0.9, 1.6)
	Unimputed	1.2 (0.9, 1.6)
Marijuana	Imputed	1.1 (0.8, 1.5)
	Unimputed	1.0 (0.7, 1.4)
Cocaine	Imputed	3.0 (1.2, 7.51)
	Unimputed	3.0 (1.3, 7.1)
Pain reliever misuse	Imputed	1.4 (0.6, 3.3)
	Unimputed	1.8 (0.7, 4.5)
Tranquilizer misuse	Imputed	17.2 (5.4, 55.0)
	Unimputed	16.7 (5.3, 53.0)

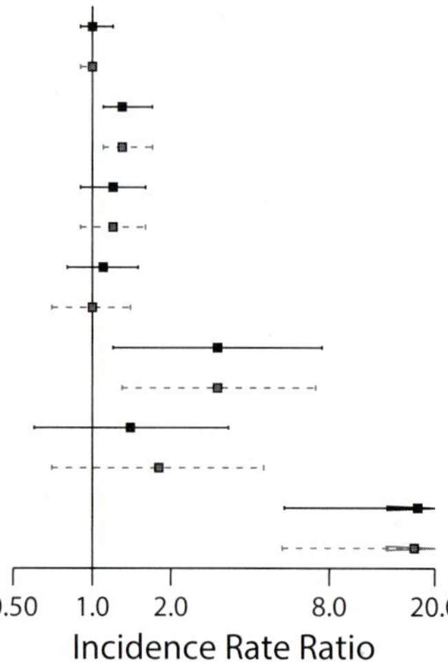

b

Past-Month Use (Y/N)		OR (95% CI)
Cigarettes	Imputed	1.2 (0.7, 2.0)
	Unimputed	1.2 (0.7, 2.0)
Alcohol	Imputed	1.0 (0.8, 1.3)
	Unimputed	1.1 (0.8, 1.4)
Binge drinking	Imputed	1.2 (0.9, 1.7)
	Unimputed	1.3 (1.0, 1.7)
Marijuana	Imputed	0.8 (0.6, 1.2)
	Unimputed	0.8 (0.6, 1.2)
Cocaine	Imputed	0.6 (0.1, 2.8)
	Unimputed	0.6 (0.1, 2.8)
Pain reliever misuse	Imputed	1.6 (0.2, 12.8)
	Unimputed	1.8 (0.2, 14.8)
Tranquilizer misuse	Imputed	4.9 (0.7, 36.2)
	Unimputed	5.1 (0.7, 37.8)

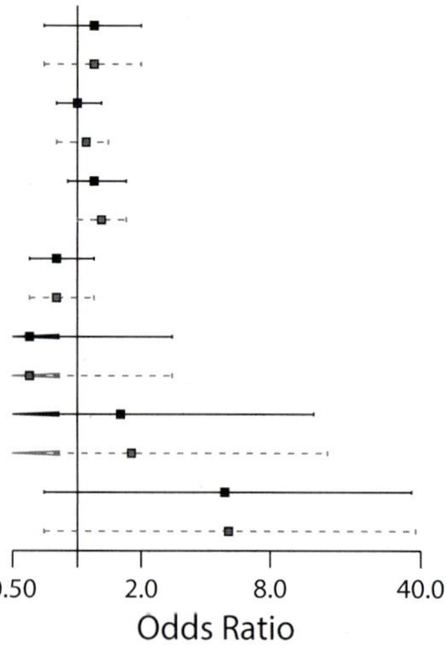

FIGURE 1— Results of Difference-in-Difference Analyses Examining the Change of the (a) Incidence and (b) Prevalence of Past-Month Substance Use or Misuse Among Asian vs White Americans Before and During the COVID-19 Pandemic: National Survey on Drug Use and Health, United States, 2016–2020

Note. CI = confidence interval; IRR = incidence rate ratio; OR = odds ratio. The sample size was n = 130 814. All models controlled for gender, age, race/ethnicity, education, employment, income, marital status, urban vs rural residence, health insurance, parental status, and self-rated health. Stimulant misuse was excluded from the analyses because of the nonparallel trend in 2016–2019 between the 2 racial groups. We estimated IRRs, ORs, and 95% CIs using the propensity score–adjusted weight. IRRs were the exponents of coefficients in multiplicative zero-inflated Poisson regression models.

use, binge drinking, marijuana use, and prescription drug misuse in 2020 compared with the previous 4 years. Finally, there were no significant differences between the 2 racial groups in the odds ratio of any substance use or misuse in 2020 compared with before. More details are presented in Tables A and B (available as a supplement to the online version of this article at http://www.ajph.org).

DISCUSSION

We investigated the change in substance use or misuse among Asian American adults in 2020 using the most recent 5-year NSDUH data. Our aim was to explore the possible population-wide impact of increased anti-Asian hate incidents. As hypothesized, we found a significant increase in the incidence rate of past-month alcohol and cocaine use and tranquilizer misuse among Asian Americans in 2020 compared with the previous 4 years relative to White Americans in 2020. In particular, the IRR of tranquilizer misuse among Asian Americans for 2020 versus 2016 to 2019 is more than 17 times the IRR among White Americans.

The first full year of the COVID-19 pandemic was 2020, when there was a noticeable increase in reported incidents of anti-Asian violence and harassment. Although anti-Asian violence is not new in US history, exposure to extensive news coverage of such incidents may have had a significant impact on the well-being of Asian Americans and those who personally experienced such incidents. Other factors, such as the stress of the pandemic itself, might have accounted for the increased substance use or misuse.

However, the fact that the increase was greater among Asian Americans than among White Americans suggests that more in-depth research is needed to test whether more types of stressors affect Asian Americans or whether there is greater susceptibility to substance use among Asian Americans. Even so, this study using DID analysis supports our hypothesis: in 2020, compared with 2016 to 2019, Asian Americans, compared with White Americans, experienced an unusual increase in incidence, but not prevalence, of stress-related substance use or misuse. Although there were no significant difference in prevalence changes, the recent increase in past-month use or misuse incidence changes of the 3 types of substances among high-risk Asian Americans relative to White Americans calls for more comprehensive assessment, identification, and treatment resources in Asian American communities. Our findings suggest that health care practitioners should record the history of using alcohol and drugs such as cocaine and tranquilizers when working with high-risk Asian American patients.

Previous research suggests that alcohol is more socially acceptable than other substances as a type of stress-coping substance in many Asian cultures.[29] However, substantial variations in alcohol consumption exist among different Asian subgroups when they experience perceived discrimination. One study found that everyday discrimination was significantly associated with increased drinking behavior among Vietnamese immigrants but not Filipino or Chinese immigrants.[30]

Factors such as acculturation, general attitudes toward drinking, family drinking history, availability of support when facing stress, and physiological reactions to alcohol ingestion contribute to diverse drinking behaviors across various groups of Asian Americans.[31] White Americans' alcohol and cocaine use declined from 2016 to 2020, which could have also contributed to the more significant differences in alcohol and cocaine use among Asian Americans in 2020 compared with White Americans. Alcohol is socially considered less harmful than illicit drug use or prescription drug misuse.[31] However, more recent data are needed to evaluate whether any high-risk Asian American subgroups have continued their increased use of alcohol since 2020. It would also be useful to explore what prevention strategies or programs Asian American communities, especially high-risk subgroups, can use to alleviate COVID-19–related stress and prevent high-risk subgroups from adopting long-term drinking behaviors.

Less is known about tranquilizer use among Asian American groups. Individuals may use tranquilizers to seek relief from heightened affective states caused by long-term stress disorders. Still, the link of stress-related dysfunction with tranquilizer use increases shared vulnerabilities and increases the likelihood of developing both psychiatric and substance use disorders.[32] The findings of this study are consistent with recent research showing an increasing trend in tranquilizer use among Asian Americans compared with use in other racial/ethnic groups.[20] However, we did not find prevalence change of tranquilizer use between the 2 racial groups. It would be worth exploring whether the increased use of tranquilizers has occurred without versus with a prescription more frequently or at higher dosages than prescribed and whether it is associated with polydrug use disorders. Our findings suggest that culturally responsive psychoeducation programs should incorporate more instruction to explain the side effects of tranquilizer misuse and how high-risk Asian Americans can access alternative stress-coping strategies.

Although we did not find any significant change in the odds of cocaine use, the change in frequency of cocaine use increased more among Asian Americans than among White Americans in 2020 compared with the change in previous years. The temporal trend in cocaine use among Asian American populations was relatively low and stable until the pandemic. However, unlike other stimulants such as methamphetamine, cocaine is perceived to be mild, less stigmatized, and less dangerous—more of a luxury recreational drug than other stimulants—especially in some young Asian American communities.[33] Therefore, during the pandemic, Asian Americans, especially those with access to cocaine, might have considered cocaine use more socially acceptable or less harmful than before. However, similar to alcohol use, cocaine use among White Americans also declined from 2016 to 2020. That also explains the more significant increase among

Asian Americans. Future research is needed to investigate the correlates of cocaine use and its patterns among Asian Americans.

Public Health Implications

The evident increase in the 3 types of substances studied among Asian Americans during the pandemic calls for attention from health and law enforcement systems and policymakers. Policymakers and those who allocate resources should focus on multilevel violence prevention efforts, such as antiracial discrimination public education programs and more security support from law enforcement, particularly in Asian communities exposed to heightened racial/ethnic harassment and violence. Asian Americans seek substance use treatment least frequently than other racial groups. Health policy and community organizations should develop culturally appropriate ways to engage Asian Americans in using socioculturally responsive substance treatment and prevention services.

Limitations

Our study had a few noteworthy limitations, which prompt suggestions for future work. First, the data in 2020 were collected mainly in quarters 1 and 4 because of the lockdown. There were fewer samples in 2020 than in previous years. Nevertheless, we adjusted our sampling weight and our propensity score weighting based on the sample size change. We also acknowledge the potential bias that may have occurred because of seasonal usage when comparing substance use in 2020 and substance use in 2016 to 2019. However, we compared the average frequency of use of each substance of interest in the past month by season for 2016 to 2019, and none of the data on substance use or misuse were significantly different across the 4 quarters of 2016 to 2019 except for binge drinking and marijuana use. Future research is needed to investigate the seasonal differences in substance use when quarter information is available.

Second, the study included a relatively large sample of Asian Americans. However, very few Asian American respondents reported using sedatives. We were unable to obtain an adjusted estimate of sedative use from the model. The low frequency of certain types of substance (e.g., tranquilizer) misuse in 2016 to 2019, especially for Asian Americans, could also threaten the accuracy of the estimation. Future research needs to continue observing the seasonal trend when such information is available. A national survey targeting Asian Americans' mental health and substance use is required to create more accurate estimates. Because of data set limitations, we were unable to disaggregate the diverse ethnic groups of Asian Americans in the United States. A broad array of ethnic, cultural, economic, geopolitical, immigration-related, and other factors contribute to heterogeneous substance use patterns between these groups.[34] Future surveys need to incorporate measurement of these critical factors so that disaggregated analysis can be conducted.

Finally, although our study suggests a higher risk of some types of substance use or misuse in 2020, it is unclear to what extent the social environment of hatred affected Asian Americans because of racial discrimination and how this relates to their substance use specifically. Additional studies are needed to collect data on racial discrimination and investigate how exposure to racial discrimination is linked with substance use among Asian Americans.

These limitations notwithstanding, this study elucidated a more significant increase in the change of some substance use or misuse among Asian Americans—whose use had been lower than that of other racial/ethnic groups—than among White Americans. Relying on the conventional approach of comparing the frequency change of use across racial/ethnic groups would leave out highly relevant groups that could benefit from prevention and intervention programs to curtail their upward use. The utility of DID analysis for this study goes beyond planning for substance use programs; it can also play an important role in other major intervention programs related to physical, mental, and behavioral health problems. AJPH

ABOUT THE AUTHORS

Yueqi Yan is with the Health Science Research Institute, University of California, Merced. Mieko Yoshihama is with the School of Social Work, University of Michigan, Ann Arbor. Jun Sung Hong is with the School of Social Work, Wayne State University, Detroit, MI, and the Department of Social Welfare, Ewha Womans University, Seoul, South Korea. Fan Jia is with the Department of Psychological Sciences, University of California, Merced.

CORRESPONDENCE

Correspondence should be sent to Yueqi Yan, PhD, Health Science Research Institute, University of California, Merced, 5200 North Lake Rd, Merced, CA 95348 (e-mail: yyan105@ucmerced.edu). Reprints can be ordered at http://www.ajph.org by clicking the "Reprints" link.

PUBLICATION INFORMATION

Full Citation: Yan Y, Yoshihama M, Hong JS, Jia F. Substance use among Asian American adults in 2016–2020: a difference-in-difference analysis of a National Survey on Drug Use and Health Data. *Am J Public Health*. 2023;113(6):671–679.

Acceptance Date: February 7, 2023.

DOI: https://doi.org/10.2105/AJPH.2023.307256

CONTRIBUTORS

Y. Yan, M. Yoshihama, and J. S. Hong conceptualized and designed the study, drafted the article, and provided administrative, technical, and material support and supervision. Y. Yan and F. Jia conducted statistical analyses. All authors contributed to data acquisition, analysis, or interpretation and critical revision of the article for important intellectual content.

CONFLICTS OF INTEREST

The authors have no potential conflicts of interest to disclose.

HUMAN PARTICIPANT PROTECTION

This study was exempt from US federal regulations for protecting human research participants because we conducted secondary data analysis using de-identified public use data from the National Survey on Drug Use and Health.

REFERENCES

1. Chen JA, Zhang E, Liu CH. Potential impact of COVID-19-related racial discrimination on the health of Asian Americans. *Am J Public Health.* 2020;110(11):1624–1627. https://doi.org/10.2105/AJPH.2020.305858
2. Lee S, Waters SF. Asians and Asian Americans' experiences of racial discrimination during the COVID-19 pandemic: impacts on health outcomes and the buffering role of social support. *Stigma Health.* 2021;6(1):70–78. https://doi.org/10.1037/sah0000275
3. Stop AAPI Hate. Two years and thousands of voices: what community-generated data tells us about anti-AAPI hate. 2022. Available at: https://stopaapihate.org/wp-content/uploads/2022/07/Stop-AAPI-Hate-Year-2-Report.pdf. Accessed March 1, 2023.
4. Jeung R, Horse AY, Popovic T, Lim R. Stop AAPI hate national report. *Ethn Stud Rep.* 2021;44(2):19–26. https://doi.org/10.1525/esr.2021.44.2.19
5. Gee GC. A multilevel analysis of the relationship between institutional and individual racial discrimination and health status. *Am J Public Health.* 2008;98(9 suppl):S48–S56. https://doi.org/10.2105/ajph.98.supplement_1.s48
6. Neblett EW Jr, Terzian M, Harriott V. From racial discrimination to substance use: the buffering effects of racial socialization. *Child Dev Perspect.* 2010;4(2):131–137. https://doi.org/10.1111/j.1750-8606.2010.00131.x
7. DeCook JR, Yoon MH. Kung flu and roof Koreans: Asian/Americans as the hated other and proxies of hating in the White imaginary. *J Hate Stud.* 2021; 17(1):119–132. https://doi.org/10.33972/jhs.199
8. Tao X, Fisher CB. Exposure to social media racial discrimination and mental health among adolescents of color. *J Youth Adolesc.* 2022;51(1):30–44. https://doi.org/10.1007/s10964-021-01514-z
9. Gerrard M, Stock ML, Roberts ME, et al. Coping with racial discrimination: the role of substance use. *Psychol Addict Behav.* 2012;26(3):550–560. https://doi.org/10.1037/a0027711
10. Gibbons FX, Pomery EA, Gerrard M. Racial discrimination and substance abuse: risk and protective factors in African American adolescents. In: Kendler KS, Thornberry TE, and Noordhuizen MMF, eds. *Handbook of Drug Use Etiology: Theory, Methods, and Empirical Findings.* Washington, DC: American Psychological Association; 2010:341–361.
11. Bennett GG, Wolin KY, Robinson EL, Fowler S, Edwards CL. Perceived racial/ethnic harassment and tobacco use among African American young adults. *Am J Public Health.* 2005;95(2):238–240. https://doi.org/10.2105/AJPH.2004.037812
12. Gibbons F, Gerrard M, Cleveland M, Wills T, Brody G. Perceived discrimination and substance use in African American parents and their children: a panel study. *J Pers Soc Psychol.* 2004; 86(4):517–529. https://doi.org/10.1037/0022-3514.86.4.517
13. Guthrie BJ, Young AM, Williams DR, Boyd CJ, Kintner EK. African American girls' smoking habits and day-to-day experiences with racial discrimination. *Nurs Res.* 2002;51(3):183–190. https://doi.org/10.1097/00006199-200205000-00007
14. Kassel JD, Stroud LR, Paronis CA. Smoking, stress, and negative affect: correlation, causation, and context across stages of smoking. *Psychol Bull.* 2003;129(2):270–304. https://doi.org/10.1037/0033-2909.129.2.270
15. Wills TA. Stress and coping factors in the epidemiology of substance use. In: Kozlowski LT, Annis HM, Cappell HD, et al., eds. *Research Advances in Alcohol and Drug Problems.* Boston, MA: Springer; 1990:215–250. https://doi.org/10.1007/978-1-4899-1669-3_7
16. Pascoe EA, Richman LS. Perceived discrimination and health: a meta-analytic review. *Psychol Bull.* 2009;135(4):531–554. https://doi.org/10.1037/a0016059
17. Sinha R. How does stress increase risk of drug abuse and relapse? *Psychopharmacology (Berl).* 2001;158(4):343–359. https://doi.org/10.1007/s002130100917
18. Otiniano Verissimo AD, Grella CE, Amaro H, Gee GC. Discrimination and substance use disorders among Latinos: the role of gender, nativity, and ethnicity. *Am J Public Health.* 2014;104(8): 1421–1428. https://doi.org/10.2105/AJPH.2014.302011
19. Hunte HER, Barry AE. Perceived discrimination and DSM-IV–based alcohol and illicit drug use disorders. *Am J Public Health.* 2012;102(12): e111–e117. https://doi.org/10.2105/AJPH.2012.300780
20. Brown P, Watts V, Hanna M, et al. Two epidemics and a pandemic: the collision of prescription drug misuse and racism during COVID-19. *J Psychoactive Drugs.* 2021;53(5):413–421. https://doi.org/10.1080/02791072.2021.1992048
21. Yoo HC, Gee GC, Lowthrop CK, Robertson J. Self-reported racial discrimination and substance use among Asian Americans in Arizona. *J Immigr Minor Health.* 2010;12(5):683–690. https://doi.org/10.1007/s10903-009-9306-z
22. Gee GC, Delva J, Takeuchi D. Relationships between self-reported unfair treatment and prescription medication use, illicit drug use, and alcohol dependence among Filipino Americans. *Am J Public Health.* 2007;97(5):933–940. https://doi.org/10.2105/AJPH.2005.075739
23. Swift SL, Glymour MM, Elfassy T, et al. Racial discrimination in medical care settings and opioid pain reliever misuse in a US cohort: 1992 to 2015. *PLoS One.* 2019;14(12):e0226490. https://doi.org/10.1371/journal.pone.0226490
24. Substance Abuse and Mental Health Services Administration. National Survey on Drug Use and Health: methodological summary and definitions. 2018. Available at: https://www.samhsa.gov/data. Accessed March 1, 2023.
25. Samples H, Stuart EA, Olfson M. Opioid use and misuse and suicidal behaviors in a nationally representative sample of US adults. *Am J Epidemiol.* 2019;188(7):1245–1253. https://doi.org/10.1093/aje/kwz061
26. Ridgeway G, Kovalchik SA, Griffin BA, Kabeto MU. Propensity score analysis with survey weighted data. *J Causal Inference.* 2015;3(2):237–249. https://doi.org/10.1515/jci-2014-0039
27. Stuart EA. Matching methods for causal inference: a review and a look forward. *Stat Sci Rev J Inst Math Stat.* 2010;25(1):1–21. https://doi.org/10.1214/09-STS313
28. Sant'Anna PHC, Zhao J. Doubly robust difference-in-differences estimators. *J Econom.* 2020;219(1): 101–122. https://doi.org/10.1016/j.jeconom.2020.06.003
29. Lui PP, Zamboanga BL. Acculturation and alcohol use among Asian Americans: a meta-analytic review. *Psychol Addict Behav.* 2018;32(2):173–186. https://doi.org/10.1037/adb0000340
30. Park SY, Anastas J, Shibusawa T, Nguyen D. The impact of acculturation and acculturative stress on alcohol use across Asian immigrant subgroups. *Subst Use Misuse.* 2014;49(8):922–931. https://doi.org/10.3109/10826084.2013.855232
31. van Amsterdam J, Opperhuizen A, Koeter M, van den Brink W. Ranking the harm of alcohol, tobacco and illicit drugs for the individual and the population. *Eur Addict Res.* 2010;16(4):202–207. https://doi.org/10.1159/000317249
32. Votaw VR, Witkiewitz K, Valeri L, Bogunovic O, McHugh RK. Nonmedical prescription sedative/tranquilizer use in alcohol and opioid use disorders. *Addict Behav.* 2019;88:48–55. https://doi.org/10.1016/j.addbeh.2018.08.010
33. Fazio A, Hunt G, Moloney M. "It's one of the better drugs to use": perceptions of cocaine use among gay and bisexual Asian American men. *Qual Health Res.* 2011;21(5):625–641. https://doi.org/10.1177/1049732310385825
34. Iwamoto DK, Kaya A, Grivel M, Clinton L. Under-researched demographics: heavy episodic drinking and alcohol-related problems among Asian Americans. *Alcohol Res.* 2016;38(1):17–25.

Rural–Urban Differences in Vaccination and Hesitancy Rates and Trust: US COVID-19 Trends and Impact Survey on a Social Media Platform, May 2021–April 2022

Sada Soorapanth, PhD, Rex Cheung, PhD, Xinzhi Zhang, MD, PhD, Ali H. Mokdad, PhD, and George A. Mensah, MD

See also Callaghan, p. 615.

Objectives. To analyze rural–urban differences in COVID-19 vaccination uptake, hesitancy, and trust in information sources in the United States.

Methods. We used data from a large survey of Facebook users. We computed the vaccination, hesitancy, and decline rates and the trust proportions among individuals hesitant toward COVID-19 information sources for rural and urban regions in each state from May 2021 to April 2022.

Results. In 48 states with adequate data, on average, two thirds of states showed statistically significant differences in monthly vaccination rates between rural and urban regions, with rural regions having a lower vaccination rate at all times. Far fewer states showed statistically significant differences when comparing monthly hesitancy and decline rates for urban versus rural regions. Doctors and health professionals received the highest level of trust. Friends and family were also among the most trusted sources in rural areas where the vaccination uptake was low.

Conclusions. Rural–urban difference in hesitancy rates among those still unvaccinated was much smaller than the rural–urban difference in vaccination rates, suggesting that access to vaccines may be another contributor to the lower vaccination rates in rural areas. (*Am J Public Health*. 2023;113(6): 680–688. https://doi.org/10.2105/AJPH.2023.307274)

AJPH June 2023, Vol 113, No. 6

Widespread vaccination is the most critical public health measure to control the COVID-19 pandemic and promote community health. However, self-reported likelihood of receiving a COVID-19 vaccine has varied over time,[1,2] and a significant proportion of US children and adults, including health care personnel, remain unvaccinated.[3] COVID-19 vaccination intent, knowledge, attitudes, and beliefs vary among different populations and geographic areas. Even among essential workers who put themselves at high risk to keep up the operations and services of local communities, only about 70% had received more than 1 vaccine dose by early June 2021, which is similar to vaccination rates among the general adult population.[4] Younger adults, non-Hispanic Black persons, and those with lower socioeconomic status were more likely to hesitate in receiving vaccination, according to the Census Bureau's Household Pulse Survey.[5,6]

Numerous studies and systematic reviews have been conducted to assess factors associated with COVID-19 vaccine hesitancy and uptake in the United States. In general, findings in these studies suggest that vaccine hesitancy is highly correlated with sociodemographic factors such as gender, race/ethnicity, age, education level, occupation, and income status as well as political preferences and religious affiliations.[5–11] Although these studies focus on the disparities in vaccination hesitancy and coverage associated with sociodemographic factors, rural–urban discrepancies in hesitancy and vaccination coverage remain incompletely understood. Studies that directly compare vaccination uptake and hesitancy in rural and urban areas at a national scale are lacking.

Published data suggest that the major determinants of vaccine hesitancy are trust in vaccine safety and effectiveness, risk perception of COVID-19 infection, and trust in government and authority.[9,12,13] Trust in science is critical in biomedical research and public health, especially among underserved populations. However, misinformation, ineffective communication, unconscious bias, and limited community engagement contribute to mistrust. Public health interventions to address misinformation and improve vaccination uptake have proven effective. For example, people who received a provider recommendation for COVID-19 vaccination were more likely to be vaccinated than were those who did not receive such a recommendation.[14] Disparities among whether people have a primary care provider could therefore lead to disparities in vaccination hesitancy and uptake.

Similar to the studies on vaccination uptake and intent, most studies on trust in COVID-19 information sources have focused on its association with sociodemographics.[1,15–17] A few focused on the role of health professionals in building trust in vaccines.[17–19] Bogart et al.[20] demonstrated the importance of having a close social network in building trust and encouraging vaccination among a sample of Black participants. There is a gap in the literature in understanding differences in trust among people living in urban and rural areas nationwide.

We investigated the rural–urban differences in vaccination uptake, hesitancy, and trust in sources of COVID-19 information to further understand variations in attitudes and potential influences to achieve better vaccination coverage for all.

METHODS

We based our study on data from the COVID-19 Trends and Impact Survey by the Delphi Group at Carnegie Mellon University, in partnership with Facebook (Delphi US CTIS).[21] The Delphi US CTIS is a large, cross-sectional survey about COVID-19 that has been delivered daily on the Facebook platform to randomly selected users in the United States since April 2020. The survey collected data on various aspects of the pandemic, such as COVID-19–like symptoms, vaccination, testing, risk behaviors, and other health and economic impacts.

The survey weights were developed in stages to adjust for sample biases. To adjust for selection and nonresponse biases, the inverse probability approach was used to create weights so that the study sample reflected the active adult population of Facebook users. To adjust for coverage bias, the weights were poststratified to match the US Census age and gender distribution for each state so that the sample reflected the general population in the United States. More details of the survey can be found in Salomon et al.[22]

Because the survey weights did not adjust for all sociodemographic factors, we took an extra step when comparing the difference in vaccination rates between urban and rural regions. Details can be found in the "Analysis" section.

Study Design

Our primary goal was to compare vaccination rates and vaccination hesitancy among rural and urban areas of the United States. Because vaccine hesitancy is mainly caused by mistrust in the COVID-19 vaccines and information people receive, our secondary goal was to compare participants' level of trust of various information sources.

We analyzed the responses to the following survey questions:

1. Have you had a COVID-19 vaccination? (Yes; No; I don't know)
2. If a vaccine to prevent COVID-19 were offered to you today, would you choose to get vaccinated? (Yes, definitely; Yes, probably; No, probably not; No, definitely not)
3. How much do you trust the following sources to provide accurate news and information about COVID-19?
   a. Doctors or other health professionals you go to for medical care
   b. Scientists and other health experts
   c. Centers for Disease Control and Prevention (CDC)
   d. Government health authorities or officials
   e. Politicians
   f. Journalists
   g. Friends and family
   h. Religious leaders

For each source, the respondent could select 1 of the following responses: "Do not trust," "Somewhat trust," or "Trust." This question was shown to all respondents.

Outcome Variables

Our study had 4 outcome measures:

1. Vaccination rate: the proportion of respondents answering "yes" to the first question. We excluded

AJPH June 2023, Vol 113, No. 6

"I don't know" responses and missing values when computing the vaccination proportion.
2. Hesitancy rate: the proportion of unvaccinated (i.e., answering "no" to the first question) respondents answering "yes, probably" or "no, probably not" to the second question.
3. Decline rate: the proportion of the unvaccinated (i.e., answering "no" to the first question) respondents answering "no, definitely not" to the second question.
4. Trust proportion: the proportion of the "trust" responses to each source in the third question. Although this question was presented to all respondents, we focused on the respondents who are unvaccinated (i.e., answered "no" to the first question) and hesitant (i.e., answered "yes, probably" or "no, probably not" to the second question).

The diagram illustrating the flow of outcome variable development is available in Figure D (available as a supplement to the online version of this article at http://www.ajph.org).

It should be noted that we defined the hesitancy rate to include unvaccinated individuals who are inclined to receive or not receive the vaccines, hence representing hesitancy both toward and against the vaccination. We believed this would more accurately represent people's uncertainty about the vaccination. This definition might be different in research in which the notion of hesitancy focuses on those who decline or are inclined not to receive the vaccines.[7,10]

Timeline

Because the eligibility for vaccines was expanded to all adults and adolescents in May 2021, we analyzed the Delphi US CTIS monthly data starting with May 2021 and extended the analysis over a 1-year period ending with April 2022.

Rural or Urban Classification

Using the zip code variable in the survey, we grouped the respondents by state. For each state, we classified the respondents' location as rural or urban by mapping the zip code to the Rural–Urban Commuting Area codes.[23] We classified the location as "urban" for Rural–Urban Commuting Area codes ranging from 1 to 3, and "rural" for those ranging from 4 to 10.

Analysis

We aggregated the data by month and computed the vaccination, hesitancy, and decline rates for each state. Because of small sample sizes, we excluded New Jersey, Rhode Island, and Washington, DC, when analyzing the vaccination rates and further excluded Alaska, Delaware, Hawaii, North Dakota, Vermont, and Wyoming when analyzing the hesitancy and decline rates.

We also stratified the rates in each state by rural versus urban areas. We plotted the rates over time and compared them between rural and urban areas. We adjusted all estimates using the survey weights provided by the Delphi Group to match the age, gender, and state profiles of the US population.[24]

To test whether the rates in rural and urban areas were significantly different, we fitted a survey-weighted generalized linear model[25] for each state. We used an individual's region (rural vs urban) as an independent variable, and we used vaccination status (or vaccine hesitancy or vaccine decline) as the dependent variable. To control for educational status (which was not adjusted by survey weights), we included education as an independent variable in the model to ensure that any differences we saw came from geographic region only. When fitting the model, any confounding factors attributed to education were absorbed by the education variable coefficient, where any remaining effect could then be attributed to rural and urban differences. We performed all computations in the statistical software R, version 3.6.3 environment, using the *svyglm* function in the *survey* package.[26] We performed the tests for all states at a significance level of $P < .05$. We applied Bonferroni correction to adjust for multiple comparisons.

For each month from May 2021 to April 2022, we also calculated the difference in the vaccination rates between urban and rural areas in each state. We then ranked the differences across 48 states (because of small sample sizes, we excluded New Jersey and Rhode Island) from the smallest (rank = 1) to the largest (rank = 48) values for each month. We then averaged the ranking values over 12 months.

To analyze trust in COVID-19 information sources, we computed the trust proportion for each source by month and plotted it over time to reveal the trend. We plotted the trust proportions across 8 sources for comparison. We also developed the plots separately for rural and urban areas to evaluate the differences.

RESULTS

The vaccination rate slowly increased over time for both urban and rural areas (Figure 1). The median vaccination rate increased, with some fluctuations, from 0.78 in May 2021 to 0.82 in April 2022 in urban areas and from

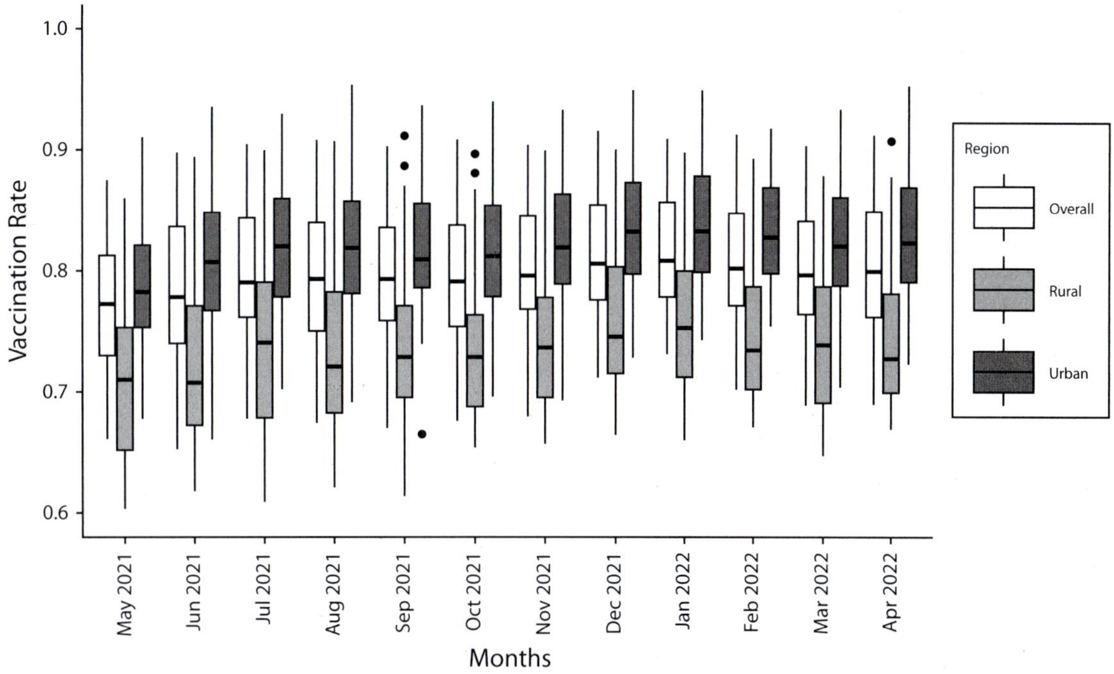

	May 2021	Jun 2021	Jul 2021	Aug 2021	Sep 2021	Oct 2021	Nov 2021	Dec 2021	Jan 2022	Feb 2022	Mar 2022	Apr 2022
Total number of responses	761 232	607 110	778 497	1 023 577	890 043	708 247	670 975	737 301	889 414	572 230	511 918	482 534
Median vaccination rate (urban)	0.78	0.80	0.82	0.82	0.81	0.81	0.82	0.83	0.83	0.83	0.82	0.82
Median vaccination rate (rural)	0.70	0.71	0.74	0.72	0.73	0.73	0.74	0.75	0.75	0.73	0.74	0.73

FIGURE 1— Five-Number Summary of Vaccination Rates Across 48 US States in a Particular Month: May 2021–April 2022

0.70 to 0.73 for the same months in rural areas. The rate was clearly lower in rural areas, and this pattern persisted across all months. The vaccination rates in rural and urban areas were significantly different in, on average, 67% of states in almost all months (range = 58%–77%; Table 1).

The states with the largest discrepancies in vaccination rates were Illinois, Ohio, Missouri, Nebraska, North Dakota, and Texas; whereas Hawaii, Mississippi, Montana, South Dakota, West Virginia, and Wyoming were among those with the lowest discrepancies. In the 6 states with the highest discrepancies, the difference in the vaccination rates between rural and urban areas was mostly more than 10% (8.3%–18.7%) for all 12 months (Figures A–D; Table A [available as a supplement to the online version of this article at http://www.ajph.org]).

Hesitancy Rate

The hesitancy rate among the unvaccinated fluctuated slightly but had a decreasing trend over time in both rural and urban areas (Figure 2). From May 21 to April 22, the median hesitancy rate decreased from 0.41 to 0.27 in the urban areas and from 0.37 to 0.25 in the rural areas. However, compared with the vaccination rate, the hesitancy rates between urban and rural areas were significantly different in, on average, only 4% (range = 0%–10%) of the 42 states investigated (Table 1).

Decline Rate

The decline rate among the unvaccinated fluctuated with an increasing trend (Figure C). From May 21 to April 22, the median decline rate increased from 0.49 to 0.70 in urban areas and from 0.54 to 0.72 in rural areas. Comparison of the trend equation of the number of unvaccinated individuals declining the vaccines and that of the number of unvaccinated individuals revealed that both variables decreased over time, but the former variable decreased more slowly than the latter. This is likely because individuals strongly opposing the vaccines did not change their opinions easily. Because the denominator (the number of unvaccinated) of the decline rate decreased faster than the numerator (the number of unvaccinated declining the vaccines), the decline rate increased over time.

Comparing the decline rates in urban and rural areas, the rates were significantly different in an average of 10%, or 4 of 42, states (range = 0%–26%; Table 1).

TABLE 1— US States Showing a Significant Difference in Vaccination Rates, Hesitancy Rates, and Decline Rates in Urban and Rural Areas: May 2021–April 2022

Month/Year	No. (%) States Showing Significant Difference		
	Vaccination Rates[a]	Hesitancy Rates[b]	Decline Rates[b]
May 2021	30 (63)	3 (7)	11 (26)
June 2021	33 (69)	4 (10)	7 (17)
July 2021	28 (58)	2 (5)	7 (17)
August 2021	35 (73)	3 (7)	9 (21)
September 2021	34 (71)	0 (0)	1 (2)
October 2021	33 (69)	1 (2)	3 (7)
November 2021	33 (69)	1 (2)	2 (5)
December 2021	29 (60)	3 (7)	4 (10)
January 2022	37 (77)	1 (2)	3 (7)
February 2022	32 (67)	0 (0)	1 (2)
March 2022	31 (65)	0 (0)	0 (0)
April 2022	31 (65)	0 (0)	1 (2)
Minimum	28 (58)	0 (0)	0 (0)
Maximum	37 (77)	4 (10)	11 (26)
Mean	32 (67)	1.5 (4)	4.1 (10)

[a]Data from 48 states (because of small sample sizes, we excluded New Jersey and Rhode Island).
[b]Data from 42 states (because of small sample sizes, we excluded New Jersey, Rhode Island, Alaska, Delaware, Hawaii, North Dakota, Vermont, and Wyoming).

Trust Proportion

Among all information sources, doctors or other health professionals had the highest proportions of trust responses, followed by scientists and other health experts, friends and families, and the CDC. Friends and families was consistently among the top 3 sources of information trusted by people living in rural areas. Politicians had the lowest proportion of trust by the public. All proportions of trust among the top sources decreased slightly between May and August with the exception of trust in friends and families, which remained relatively stable over time (Figure 3).

DISCUSSION

We analyzed a large national public health survey that surveyed a stratified random sampling of Facebook users from diverse socioeconomic statuses and geographic areas. We showed that although the overall vaccination rate increased over time, the vaccination rates between rural and urban regions were significantly different in most states, and the rural regions had lower vaccination rates at all times. However, when comparing hesitancy rates among unvaccinated persons in rural versus urban areas, there were no significant differences in most states, implying that, among those still not vaccinated, the receptiveness of people to vaccines may not be much different between rural and urban areas in most states. We reran the analysis with the definition of hesitancy used in other literature (i.e., focusing only on people who do not want to receive the vaccines).[7,10] Although this changed the numerical results, it did not change our conclusion qualitatively.

The rural–urban differences in vaccination coverage have already been reported in Saelee et al.[27] However, we not only analyzed the vaccination uptake but further investigated the intent or hesitancy, providing a more comprehensive understanding of rural–urban differences with regard to the COVID-19 vaccination.

Our key finding that the vaccination rates were significantly different in rural and urban areas but the hesitancy rates (among those still unvaccinated) were not has an important implication. It suggests that access to the vaccines could contribute to the lower vaccination rates in rural regions. Thus, COVID-19 vaccination differences may be one more manifestation of the long-standing and more general problem of health care access in the United States. As of March 31, 2022, 5134 of 7832 (65.6%) designated primary care health professional shortage areas are in rural areas.[28] The North Carolina Rural Health Research and Policy Analysis Center also reported a fluctuation but an overall increasing trend in hospital closures in rural areas since 2010.[29] According to a Pew Research Center survey conducted in 2018, 23% of Americans in rural areas say access to good doctors and hospitals is a major problem in their community compared with 18% of urbanites and 9% of suburbanites.[30]

Our rural–urban vaccination rate discrepancy analysis revealed the 6 states with the largest discrepancies, ranging from approximately 10% to 19%. The map in Figure B shows that most of these states are located in the Midwest. Except for North Dakota, which could not be evaluated because of its small sample size, the rural–urban hesitancy rates were not significantly different in

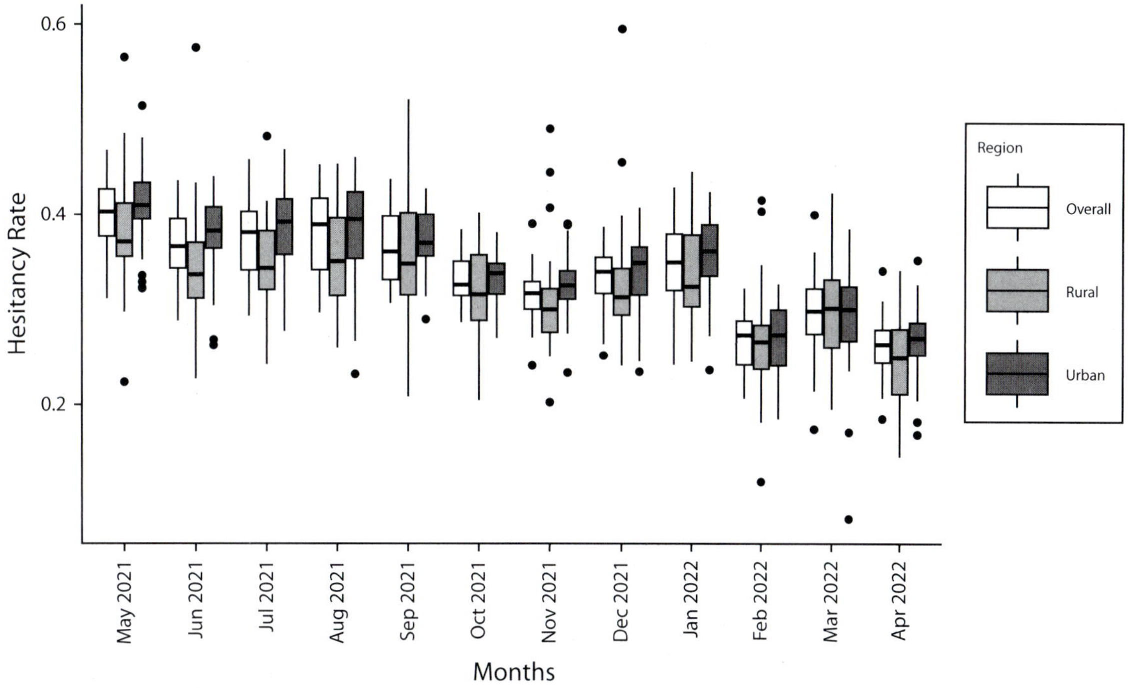

	May 2021	Jun 2021	Jul 2021	Aug 2021	Sep 2021	Oct 2021	Nov 2021	Dec 2021	Jan 2022	Feb 2022	Mar 2022	Apr 2022
Total number of responses	137 116	97 579	117 130	156 367	133 454	106 410	97 202	99 783	121 533	73 602	80 317	66 759
Median hesitancy rate (urban)	0.41	0.38	0.39	0.40	0.37	0.34	0.33	0.35	0.37	0.28	0.30	0.27
Median hesitancy rate (rural)	0.37	0.34	0.35	0.36	0.35	0.32	0.30	0.32	0.33	0.27	0.31	0.25

FIGURE 2— **Five-Number Summary of Hesitancy Rates Across 42 US States in a Particular Month: May 2021–April 2022**

most months. No definite conclusion can be drawn from these data regarding this phenomenon, and further investigation should be conducted with other data sources to understand the cause of this discrepancy.

Lastly, our results from the analysis of trust in information sources indicate that doctors and health professions received the highest level of trust, followed by scientists and other health experts. This conclusion holds for both rural and urban areas. Friends and family received the next highest level among the respondents in rural areas where the vaccination uptake remained low. These findings confirm the results in other studies, although they were conducted in a smaller sample size or focused on particular subpopulations.[19,20] Our results are based on data from nationwide and diverse populations, making the findings more generalizable.

In general, poor health literacy has been a key barrier to seeking care. The hesitancy toward and misunderstanding about COVID-19 vaccines and mistrust in science highlight this challenge. A systematic review of 44 studies[31] reported a relationship between reading ability and utilization of health care services, health outcomes, and disparities in health care service utilization and health outcomes. Studies in the review found that patients with low reading ability were more likely to not receive basic services such as influenza and pneumococcal immunization and cancer screenings. Rural areas are still behind urban areas in their literacy rates. According to the report by Pew Research Center,[30] 35% of urban residents have college degrees compared with 19% in rural counties.

These findings emphasize the need for public health programs that can engage local communities with their health care providers, community-based organizations, and other community partners to provide accurate, science-based information, reduce vaccine hesitancy, and promote vaccination uptake. Our analysis also shows that the hesitancy rate among the unvaccinated has had a decreasing trend over time in both rural and urban areas, which may largely be attributable to public health programs such as the National Institutes of Health–funded Community Engagement Alliance Against COVID-19 Disparities (https://COVID19community.nih.gov), RADx–Underserved Populations

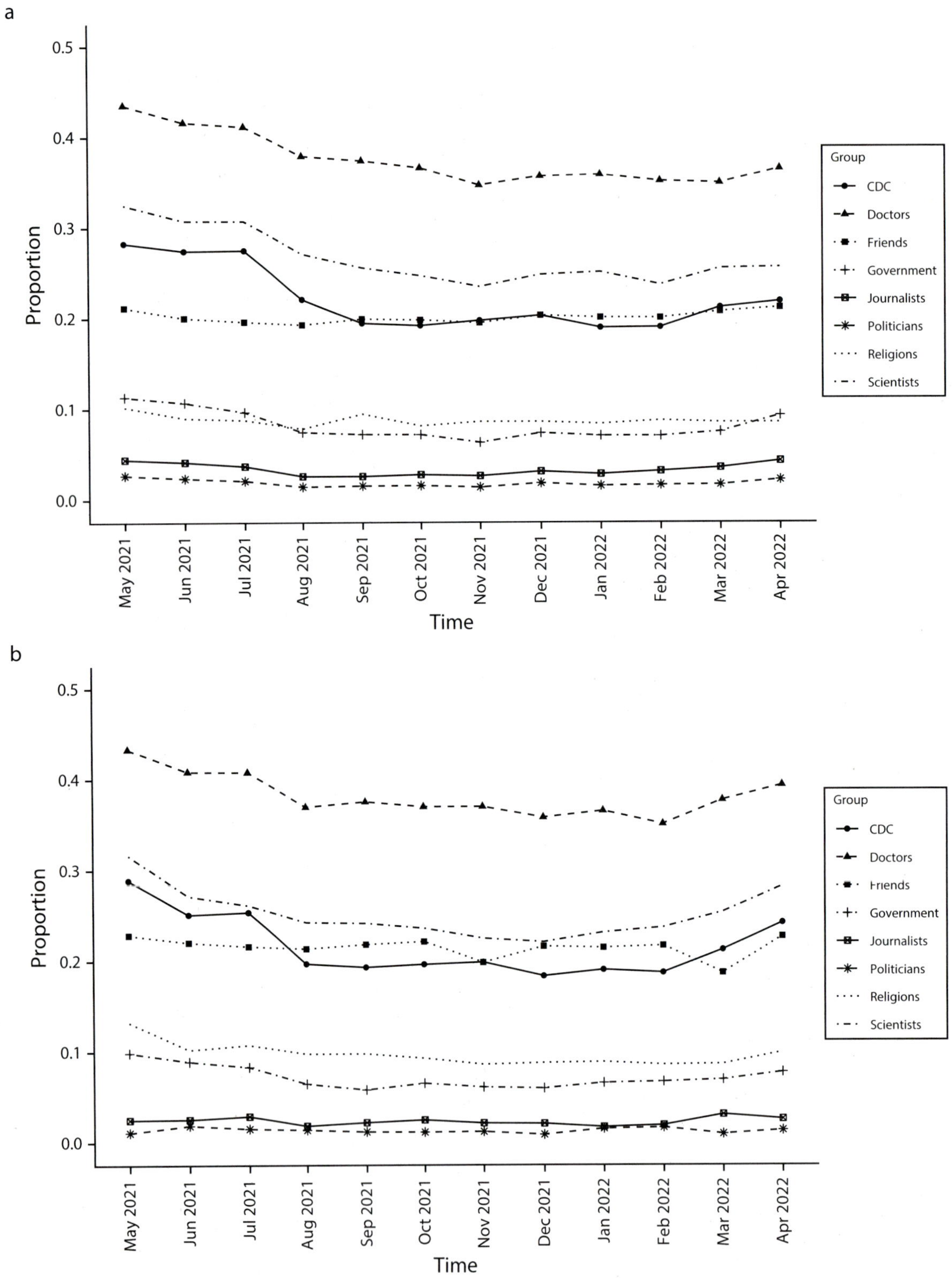

FIGURE 3— Proportions of Trust Responses Among Survey Respondents Who Are Unvaccinated and Hesitate to Be Vaccinated in (a) Urban and (b) Rural Areas: United States, May 2021–April 2022

Note. CDC = Centers for Disease Control and Prevention.

(https://radx-up.org), and the COVID-19 Prevention Network (https://www.coronaviruspreventionnetwork.org). Major academic health centers, rural health centers, and community health workers can also play important roles in reducing rural–urban health disparities.

The rural–urban differences in COVID-19 vaccination shown in this study and in COVID-19–related health outcomes reported elsewhere should not come as a surprise. The pandemic has accentuated the underlying problems that have long existed in rural communities, in particular, unequal access to care because of hospital closures, health care personnel shortages, misinformation and mistrust, and insufficient communication outreach. Although some progress has been made to mediate the issues, including building community partnership programs and expanding the use of health innovations such as telemedicine, a more comprehensive approach is necessary.

Limitations

This study has several limitations. First, the results rely on the accuracy of the survey reporting. Trolling responses exist in surveys.[32] Second, the survey may contain repeated respondents. According to the survey description,[21] each respondent was sampled in the survey every 1 to 6 months. Therefore, our analyses were conducted on a monthly basis to ensure the uniqueness of the respondents. Although it was unlikely that the respondents would take the same survey repeatedly from month to month, because we did not know to what extent the survey contained repeated respondents across months, we chose a rather conservative approach to compare the rural–urban outcomes in each month only.

Third, because of limited information and sample sizes in the current survey data, we were unable to address rurality among different rural areas by states and its potential impact on access to COVID-19 vaccination and migration strategies. Although a town outside Atlanta, Georgia, and a small frontier city in eastern Colorado may both be defined as "rural," those populations may differ substantially.

Fourth, the language coverage of the survey and its impact on the representation of minorities in rural populations have not been evaluated. However, the survey was translated into Spanish, Chinese, French, Brazilian Portuguese, and Vietnamese. According to the 2020 census, 76.0% of rural populations are non-Hispanic White, 9.0% are Hispanic, 7.7% are Black, 2.5% are Native American/other race, 1.0% are Asian, and 3.9% are non-Hispanic multiracial.[33] Therefore, the languages covered by the survey should account for the majority of rural populations. Lastly, although we applied the survey weights to adjust for sampling, nonresponse, and coverage biases, there are still factors that have not been accounted for and could affect our results. For example, the weights do not account for income and political affiliation or philosophy. These factors could affect the ability to access the vaccines and attitudes toward vaccination, hence affecting the validity of our conclusion.

Conclusions and Public Health Implications

The rural–urban difference in hesitancy rates among those still unvaccinated was much smaller than the rural–urban difference in vaccination rates, suggesting that access to vaccines may be another contributor to the lower vaccination rates in rural areas. In both rural and urban areas, trusted sources of COVID-19 information exist and can play a crucial role in addressing misinformation and distrust. Active community engagement and outreach to rural communities to improve awareness and access to vaccines is warranted. AJPH

ABOUT THE AUTHORS

Sada Soorapanth and Rex Cheung are with the Department of Decision Sciences, Lam Family College of Business, San Francisco State University, San Francisco, CA. Xinzhi Zhang and George A. Mensah are with the Center for Translation Research and Implementation Science, National Heart, Lung, and Blood Institute, National Institutes of Health, Bethesda, MD. Ali H. Mokdad is with the Institute for Health Metrics and Evaluation and the Department of Health Metrics Sciences, School of Medicine, University of Washington, Seattle.

CORRESPONDENCE

Correspondence should be sent to Sada Soorapanth, PhD, Department of Decision Sciences, Lam Family College of Business, San Francisco State University, 1600 Holloway Ave, San Francisco, CA 94132 (e-mail: sada@sfsu.edu). Reprints can be ordered at http://www.ajph.org by clicking the "Reprints" link.

PUBLICATION INFORMATION

Full Citation: Soorapanth S, Cheung R, Zhang X, Mokdad AH, Mensah GA. Rural–urban differences in vaccination and hesitancy rates and trust: US COVID-19 trends and impact survey on a social media platform, May 2021–April 2022. *Am J Public Health*. 2023;113(6):680–688.

Acceptance Date: February 16, 2023.

DOI: https://doi.org/10.2105/AJPH.2023.307274

CONTRIBUTORS

All authors were involved in all steps of this work, including planning, analysis, interpreting the results, and making conclusions. All reviewed and edited the article at all phases.

ACKNOWLEDGMENTS

We thank the Delphi Group at Carnegie Mellon University and Facebook for allowing us to use their data for this analysis. We also thank the Lam Family College of Business and the Office of Research and Sponsored Programs at San Francisco State University for their support.

Note. The contents and views expressed in this article are those of the authors and do not necessarily reflect the official views of the National Heart, Lung, and Blood Institute, the National Institutes of Health, the US government, or the affiliated institutions.

CONFLICTS OF INTEREST

The authors do not have any conflicts of interest to disclose.

HUMAN PARTICIPANT PROTECTION

We used information for which consent was not required and data from survey participants whose identity cannot be obtained by the investigators; therefore, this study did not require institutional review board approval.

REFERENCES

1. Szilagyi PG, Thomas K, Shah MD, et al. National trends in the US public's likelihood of getting a COVID-19 vaccine—April 1 to December 8, 2020. *JAMA.* 2021;325(4):396–398. https://doi.org/10.1001/jama.2020.26419
2. Nguyen KH, Nguyen K, Geddes M, Allen JD, Corlin L. Trends in COVID-19 vaccination receipt and intention to vaccinate, United States, April to August, 2021. *Am J Infect Control.* 2022;50(6):699–703. https://doi.org/10.1016/j.ajic.2021.12.022
3. Razzaghi H, Masalovich S, Srivastav A, et al. COVID-19 vaccination and intent among healthcare personnel, US. *Am J Prev Med.* 2022;62(5):705–715. https://doi.org/10.1016/j.amepre.2021.11.001
4. Nguyen KH, Yankey D, Coy KC, et al. COVID-19 vaccination coverage, intent, knowledge, attitudes, and beliefs among essential workers, United States. *Emerg Infect Dis.* 2021;27(11):2908–2913. https://doi.org/10.3201/eid2711.211557
5. Nguyen KH, Nguyen K, Corlin L, Allen JD, Chung M. Changes in COVID-19 vaccination receipt and intention to vaccinate by socioeconomic characteristics and geographic area, United States, January 6–March 29, 2021. *Ann Med.* 2021;53(1):1419–1428. https://doi.org/10.1080/07853890.2021.1957998
6. Nguyen KH, Anneser E, Toppo A, Allen JD, Scott Parott J, Corlin L. Disparities in national and state estimates of COVID-19 vaccination receipt and intent to vaccinate by race/ethnicity, income, and age group among adults ≥ 18 years, United States. *Vaccine.* 2022;40(1):107–113. https://doi.org/10.1016/j.vaccine.2021.11.040
7. Khubchandani J, Sharma S, Price JH, Wiblishauser MJ, Sharma M, Webb FJ. COVID-19 vaccination hesitancy in the United States: a rapid national assessment. *J Community Health.* 2021;46(2):270–277. https://doi.org/10.1007/s10900-020-00958-x
8. Yasmin F, Najeeb H, Moeed A, et al. COVID-19 vaccine hesitancy in the United States: a systematic review. *Front Public Health.* 2021;9:770985. https://doi.org/10.3389/fpubh.2021.770985
9. Joshi A, Kaur M, Kaur R, Grover A, Nash D, El-Mohandes A. Predictors of COVID-19 vaccine acceptance, intention, and hesitancy: a scoping review. *Front Public Health.* 2021;9:698111. https://doi.org/10.3389/fpubh.2021.698111
10. King WC, Rubinstein M, Reinhart A, Mejia R. Time trends, factors associated with, and reasons for COVID-19 vaccine hesitancy: a massive online survey of US adults from January–May 2021. *PLoS One.* 2021;16(12):e0260731. https://doi.org/10.1371/journal.pone.0260731
11. Levin J, Bradshaw M. Determinants of COVID-19 skepticism and SARS-CoV-2 vaccine hesitancy: findings from a national population survey of US adults. *BMC Public Health.* 2022;22(1):1047. https://doi.org/10.1186/s12889-022-13477-2
12. Thunström L, Ashworth M, Finnoff D, Newbold SC. Hesitancy toward a COVID-19 vaccine. *EcoHealth.* 2021;18(1):44–60. https://doi.org/10.1007/s10393-021-01524-0
13. Viswanath K, Bekalu M, Dhawan D, Pinnamaneni R, Lang J, McLoud R. Individual and social determinants of COVID-19 vaccine uptake. *BMC Public Health.* 2021;21(1):818. https://doi.org/10.1186/s12889-021-10862-1
14. Centers for Disease Control and Prevention. Report of health care provider recommendation for COVID-19 vaccination among adults, by recipient COVID-19 vaccination status and attitudes—United States, April–September 2021. *MMWR Morb Mortal Wkly Rep.* 2021;70(50):1723–1730. https://doi.org/10.15585/mmwr.mm7050a1
15. Purvis RS, Hallgren E, Moore RA, et al. Trusted sources of COVID-19 vaccine information among hesitant adopters in the United States. *Vaccines (Basel).* 2021;9(12):1418. https://doi.org/10.3390/vaccines9121418
16. Bagasra AB, Doan S, Allen CT. Racial differences in institutional trust and COVID-19 vaccine hesitancy and refusal. *BMC Public Health.* 2021;21(1):2104. https://doi.org/10.1186/s12889-021-12195-5
17. Brauer E, Choi K, Chang J, et al. Health care providers' trusted sources for information about COVID-19 vaccines: mixed methods study. *JMIR Infodemiology.* 2021;1(1):e33330. https://doi.org/10.2196/33330
18. Wang Y, Liu Y. Multilevel determinants of COVID-19 vaccination hesitancy in the United States: a rapid systematic review. *Prev Med Rep.* 2021;25:101673. https://doi.org/10.1016/j.pmedr.2021.101673
19. Shen AK, Tan ASL. Trust, influence, and community: why pharmacists and pharmacies are central for addressing vaccine hesitancy. *J Am Pharm Assoc (2003).* 2022;62(1):305–308. doi: 10.1016/j.japh.2021.10.001
20. Bogart LM, Dong L, Gandhi P, et al. COVID-19 vaccine intentions and mistrust in a national sample of Black Americans. *J Natl Med Assoc.* 2022;113(6):599–611. https://doi.org/10.1016/j.jnma.2021.05.011
21. Carnegie Mellon University, Delphi Research Group. COVID-19 Trends and Impact Survey. Available at: https://cmu-delphi.github.io/delphi-epidata/symptom-survey/#covid-19-trends-and-impact-survey. Accessed March 21, 2023.
22. Salomon JA, Reinhart A, Bilinski A, et al. The US COVID-19 Trends and Impact Survey: continuous real-time measurement of COVID-19 symptoms, risks, protective behaviors, testing, and vaccination. *Proc Natl Acad Sci USA.* 2021;118(51):e2111454118. https://doi.org/10.1073/pnas.2111454118
23. US Department of Agriculture, Economic Research Service. Rural–urban commuting area codes. August 17, 2020. Available at: https://www.ers.usda.gov/data-products/rural-urban-commuting-area-codes. Accessed March 21, 2023.
24. Meta. User guide for the COVID-19 trends and impact survey weights. May 10, 2022. Available at: https://dataforgood.facebook.com/dfg/resources/user-guide-for-ctis-weights. Accessed March 21, 2023.
25. Lumley T, Scott A. Fitting regression models to survey data. *Stat Sci.* 2017;32(2):265–278. https://doi.org/10.1214/16-STS605
26. Lumley T. Survey: analysis of complex survey samples. 2020. R package version 4.0 [computer program]. Available at: https://cran.r-project.org/web/packages/survey/index.html. Accessed March 28, 2023.
27. Centers for Disease Control and Prevention. Disparities in COVID-19 vaccination coverage between urban and rural counties—United States, December 14, 2020–January 31, 2022. *MMWR Morb Mortal Wkly Rep.* 2022;71(9):335–340. https://doi.org/10.15585/mmwr.mm7109a2
28. Health Resources and Services Administration. Designated health professional shortage areas statistics. March 31 2022. Available at: https://data.hrsa.gov/Default/GenerateHPSAQuarterlyReport. Accessed June 24, 2022.
29. University of North Carolina, Rural Health Research and Policy Analysis Center. Rural hospital closures. Available at: http://www.shepscenter.unc.edu/programs-projects/rural-health/rural-hospital-closures. Accessed June 24, 2022.
30. Pew Research Center. What unites and divides urban, suburban and rural communities. May 2018. Available at: https://www.pewresearch.org/social-trends/2018/05/22/views-of-problems-facing-urban-suburban-and-rural-communities. Accessed March 21, 2023.
31. Dewalt DA, Berkman ND, Sheridan S, Lohr KN, Pignone MP. Literacy and health outcomes: a systematic review of the literature. *J Gen Intern Med.* 2004;19(12):1228–1239. https://doi.org/10.1111/j.1525-1497.2004.40153.x
32. Lopez J, Hillygus DS. Why so serious? Survey trolls and misinformation. March 14, 2018. Available at: https://doi.org/10.2139/ssrn.3131087. Accessed March 21, 2023.
33. Johnson KM, Lichter D. Growing racial diversity in rural America: results from the 2020 Census. Available at: https://scholars.unh.edu/carsey/449. Accessed March 21, 2023.

Competencies, Training Needs, and Turnover Among Rural Compared With Urban Local Public Health Practitioners: 2021 Public Health Workforce Interests and Needs Survey

Paula M. Kett, RN, PhD, MPH, Betty Bekemeier, RN, PhD, MPH, Davis G. Patterson, PhD, and Kay Schaffer, MPH

See also Harris, p. 607.

Objectives. To compare rural versus urban local public health workforce competencies and training needs, COVID-19 impact, and turnover risk.

Methods. Using the 2021 Public Health Workforce Interest and Needs Survey, we examined the association between local public health agency rural versus urban location in the United States (n = 29 751) and individual local public health staff reports of skill proficiencies, training needs, turnover risk, experiences of bullying due to work as a public health professional, and posttraumatic stress disorder symptoms attributable to COVID-19.

Results. Rural staff had higher odds than urban staff of reporting proficiencies in community engagement, cross-sectoral partnerships, and systems and strategic thinking as well as training needs in data-based decision-making and in diversity, equity, and inclusion. Rural staff were also more likely than urban staff to report leaving because of stress, experiences of bullying, and avoiding situations that made them think about COVID-19.

Conclusions. Our findings demonstrate that rural staff have unique competencies and training needs but also experience significant stress.

Public Health Implications. Our findings provide the opportunity to accurately target rural workforce development trainings and illustrate the need to address reported stress and experiences of bullying.
(*Am J Public Health*. 2023;113(6):689–699. https://doi.org/10.2105/AJPH.2023.307273)

AJPH June 2023, Vol 113, No. 6

The COVID-19 pandemic has placed considerable strain on the US public health workforce. High turnover of local health department (LHD) personnel has occurred, creating concern about workforce needs and capacity.[1,2] These circumstances have compounded stressors that LHDs faced before the pandemic, including inadequate funding and support, insufficient staffing, and gaps in competencies for promoting community health.[3–5] This strain has been particularly severe among rural LHDs through an historical lack of investment and limited workforce capacity relative to their urban counterparts.[6] Rural LHDs provide essential community services, operating as safety net providers and engaging in population-based services. A deeper understanding of rural LHD workforce assets and needs is critical to providing effective support for strengthening our rural public health systems.[7,8]

The public health workforce—including nurses, environmental health professionals, epidemiologists, and others—engages in population-focused interventions, individual-level direct services, and policy development to protect the public's health and reduce disparities.[9] As public health systems have shifted efforts toward population-based services, required workforce competencies have also shifted: skills are needed in community engagement, cross-sectoral partnerships, systems thinking, and policy development, along with capacity to promote health equity.[10–12] The pandemic further highlighted needs for data science and evaluation skills, which may be underdeveloped among rural LHDs.[7,13] Research is needed to understand rural workforce competencies and gaps as part of supporting provision of more population-based services.[14]

Rural LHD personnel confront unique challenges in improving population health in communities with limited resources. Rural LHDs and their staff, compared with their urban neighbors, are the least well-resourced component of our public health systems, with less funding, fewer staff, and less training because funding often depends, in part, on an area's tax base and local wealth.[6] Rural LHDs also have smaller networks of organizations with whom to partner, further limiting their capacity, yet they serve communities with higher rates of risky behaviors and poor health outcomes than urban areas.[8,15] Furthermore, rural LHDs tend to rely on clinical service revenue, complicating their ability to transition to providing more population-based services.[8] Larger threats to LHD workforce supply and development may also exist, including geographical differences in staff turnover risk and the impact of COVID-19.

Previous LHD workforce research has been largely limited to medium-sized and large LHDs and overall has lacked rural–urban comparisons because of data limitations.[4,16–19] For example, initial analyses from the 2021 Public Health Workforce Interest and Needs Survey (PH WINS) show that approximately 27% of respondents intended to leave their agency in the next year; it is unknown, however, how this differs between rural and urban staff.[1] One study of local competency gaps examined rural–urban differences but focused on 1 state.[16] Other studies exploring competencies and training needs have centered on or included state public health employees without sufficient attention to local jurisdictions.[20–23] Furthermore, most studies exploring workforce competencies, training needs, intent to leave, and other outcomes using PH WINS have not incorporated additional LHD organizational factors such as leadership background (e.g., physician, nurse) or public health workforce supply. In this study, we aimed to fill these gaps by comparing rural versus urban LHD workforce competencies and training needs, COVID-19 impact, and turnover risk to enable targeted investments, training, and support for the rural LHD workforce to serve their communities.

METHODS

We compiled a national data set including individual-level LHD staff competencies, training needs, COVID-19 experiences, and staff turnover risk as well as LHD characteristics and county-level demographics. Individual-level staff variables came from the 2021 PH WINS, a nationally representative survey of individual state and local governmental public health staff administered by the de Beaumont Foundation and the Association of State and Territorial Health Officials.[1] The 2021 PH WINS was sent to 137 446 nonsupervisors (tier 1 staff), supervisors and managers (tier 2 staff), and executives (tier 3 staff) in 47 state health departments; 29 big city health departments; 497 LHDs in states with centralized, shared, or mixed public health governance; and 259 decentralized LHDs. The response rate for the national sample was 35% (n = 44 732). The same survey included respondents from the US Department of Health and Human Services Regions 5 (Illinois, Indiana, Michigan, Minnesota, Ohio, and Wisconsin) and 10 (Alaska, Idaho, Oregon, and Washington) in the pilot program "PH WINS for All." This pilot program collected PH WINS data through a census of all LHDs in these regions, including LHDs that had fewer than 25 full-time equivalent employees (FTEs), that served populations of fewer than 25 000, or both.[24] These small LHDs had not been included previously in PH WINS. The methods for this census survey portion of PH WINS are described elsewhere,[24] but these PH WINS data representing staff serving small population sizes are generally rural communities. Data on LHD organizational characteristics came from the 2019 National Profile of Local Health Departments Survey (hereafter called Profile) conducted by the National Association of County and City Health Officials (NACCHO). We derived county demographic data from the 2020 Area Health Resource File (AHRF). We linked PH WINS and Profile data using NACCHO identifiers and AHRF data via county-level Federal Information Processing System (FIPS) codes.

Our data set included only LHD respondents to PH WINS (not state-level respondents). The final sample consisted of 29 751 tier 1–3 staff respondents from 742 LHDs.

Measures

Independent variables. The key independent variable was the rural–urban classification of respondents' LHDs. "Urban" was the reference category in all regression analyses. We classified LHDs as rural or urban using 2019 Profile urban–rural designations for LHDs, based on the National Center for Health Statistics Urban-Rural Classification scheme and frontier and remote area (FAR) codes.[14] LHD characteristics included were whether the LHD director was a clinician (physician, nurse, dentist, veterinarian), whether the LHD was accredited by the Public Health Accreditation Board, and FTEs per 1000 population.[25,26]

Individual-level LHD staff indicators included public health practice tenure (0–5 years, > 5 years) and education level (master's degree or higher, less than a master's). County-level characteristics of the LHD's jurisdiction included percentages of population unemployed, persons in poverty, and persons older than 25 years with less than a high school diploma, as well as percentages of Black, Hispanic, and American Indian/Alaska Native populations.

We examined other variables included in past PH WINS analyses and other research, such as whether an agency's local board of health had policymaking authority and LHD staff respondents' race, ethnicity, and age. Because their inclusion did not substantially affect our results, these variables were not retained in final models.

Dependent variables. We examined dependent variables measuring skills, training needs, COVID-19 impact, and turnover risk. Tier 1, 2, and 3 respondents reported proficiency in and importance of skills in their day-to-day work across 9 domains (e.g., "Data-Based Decision-Making" and "Effective Communication"; Figure 1). Skills and training needs were measured by staff tiers; all other outcomes were examined across all staff. Because of the small number of tier 3 respondents and the similar skills listed for tiers 2 and 3, we combined these tiers for each tier-based outcome ("tier 2/3").

Likert scales measured skill proficiency (0 = not applicable, 1 = unable to perform, 2 = beginner, 3 = proficient, 4 = expert) and importance (1 = not important, 2 = somewhat unimportant, 3 = somewhat important, 4 = very important). We transformed skill area variables (23 skills for tier 1 and 24 for tier 2/3) into binary variables (0 = unable to perform or beginner and 1 = proficient or expert). We excluded "not applicable" responses, which ranged from 5% to 15% depending on skill area. We defined "training need" to mean when respondents reported skills as "somewhat important" or "very important" to their day-to-day work and they reported their competency level for those skills as "unable to perform" or "beginner," similar to how previous studies have defined training needs.[18,19,23] We transformed training needs into binary variables (1 = high importance and low skill and 0 = all other combinations, e.g., high importance and high skill).

We assessed turnover risk by the question, "Are you considering leaving your organization in the next year?" Those reporting intentions to leave were asked to select among reasons. A separate question asked whether COVID-19 influenced their intention to leave. We examined turnover risk and influence of COVID-19 using binary variables, including intent to leave in the next year (excluding retirement), reasons for intending to leave, and feeling bullied, threatened, or harassed.

Two additional questions examined COVID-19 impact in terms of COVID-19 posttraumatic stress disorder (PTSD) symptoms and experiences of being bullied or harassed due to being a public health professional.[1] Measures of PTSD symptoms used survey items from an existing primary care PTSD screen.[1]

Analysis

We computed descriptive statistics and used the χ^2 test for bivariate analyses, evaluating significance at $P < .01$. We used multivariable logistic regression analysis to assess odds ratios of skill proficiency, training needs, turnover risk, and impact of COVID-19 for rural versus urban staff; skill proficiency and training needs were analyzed in separate tier 1 and tier 2/3 models. We constructed models using a phased approach, starting with bivariate associations between each outcome and rural–urban location followed by other staff, organizational, and community characteristics. We present fully adjusted models, displaying coefficients for all analyses, along with 95% confidence intervals, in exponentiated form.

Because our full PH WINS participant sample included census survey respondents from LHDs serving small populations or with small staffs, we did not use the balanced repeated replication weights included with the survey; inclusion of weights would have decreased our rural sample and removed small LHDs.[24,27] Approximately 5000 PH WINS respondents did not have corresponding LHD Profile data. The proportions of rural and urban respondents missing Profile data were relatively similar (rural: 827 [20%]; urban: 4011 [16%]). We analyzed models with and

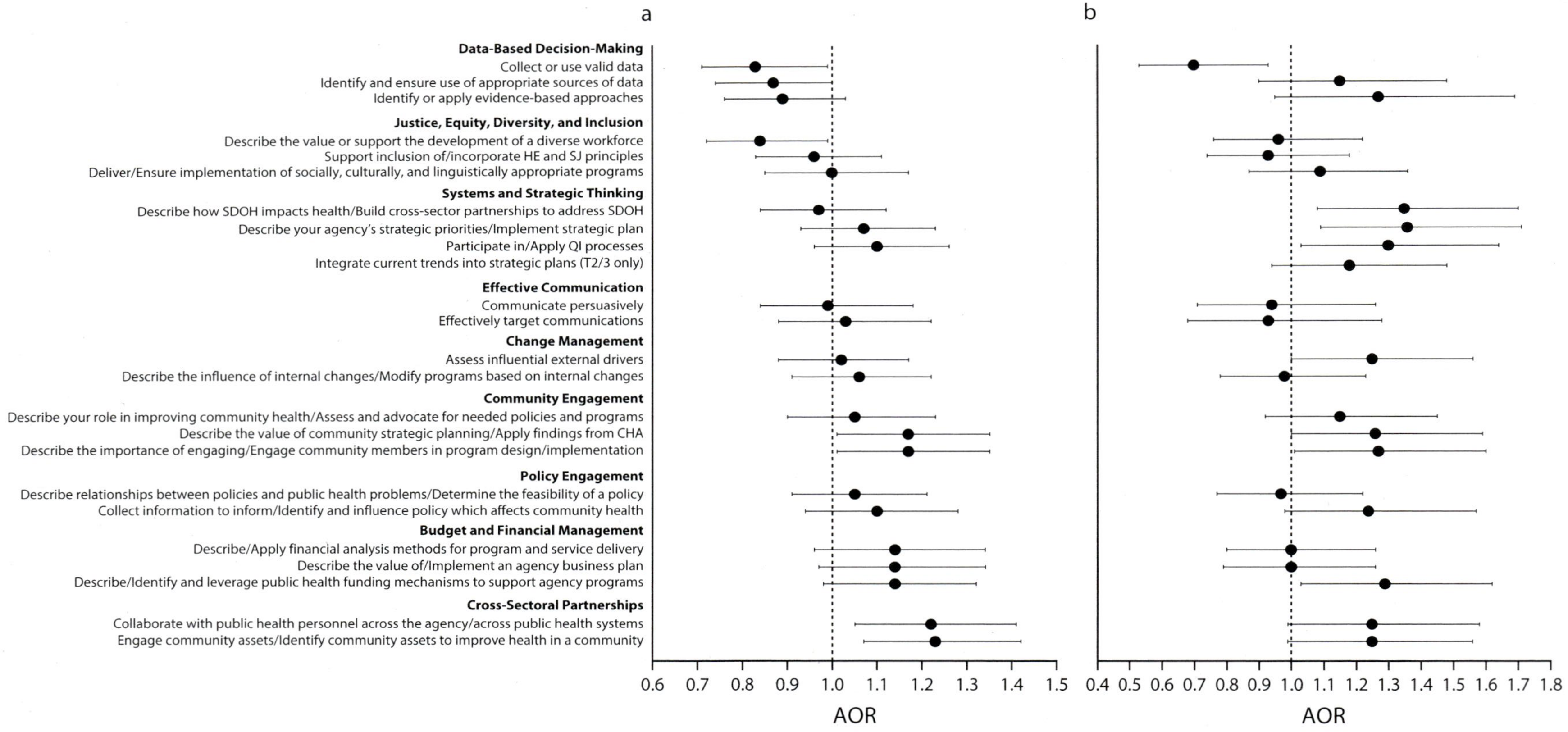

FIGURE 1— **Rural vs Urban Skill Proficiency Among Nonsupervisors and Supervisors/Executives in Local Health Departments by (a) Tier 1 Skill Proficiency and (b) Tier 2/3 Skill Proficiency: United States, 2021**

Note. AOR = adjusted odds ratio; CHA = community health assessment; HE = health equity; QI = quality improvement; SDOH = social determinants of health; SJ = social justice. All results of the logistic regression are presented in their exponentiated form as odds ratios with urban as the reference category; AOR = 1.0 is not statistically significant. All outcomes are adjusted for local health department organizational variables (clinician-led, accreditation, full-time equivalent employees per 1000 population), staff variables (tenure, education level), and community-level variables (% unemployed, % in poverty, % older than 25 years with < high school diploma, % Black population, % Hispanic population, and % American Indian/Alaska Native population). Numerical values are available in Table C (available as a supplement to the online version of this article at http://www.ajph.org). Skill names are abbreviated; full names are available in online Table C. Skills with a "/" indicate tier 1 and tier 2/3 wording; tier 2/3 wording follows the "/."

without these respondents; results were not substantially different, and we included respondents with missing Profile data in our analyses. Sensitivity testing also included analyses using multilevel modeling techniques to account for clustering within and between LHDs; clustering at this level accounted for a small level of variance, with outcomes similar to those in the logistic regression analyses.

RESULTS

Most respondents self-identified as female, were 31 to 50 years old, had bachelor's or lower degrees, and had worked in public health for 5 or more years (Table 1). In rural areas, 75% of respondents self-identified as White, a much larger proportion than urban staff (48%). Staffing relative to population size was higher in rural LHDs (0.9 FTEs per 1000 population) compared with urban LHDs (0.6 FTEs per 1000 population). More urban than rural LHDs were accredited (64% vs 32%). On average, a higher percentage of urban versus rural populations were at or below the federal poverty level according to US Census criteria (15% vs 12%), with lower median household incomes ($51 200 vs $65 000) and lower percentages identifying as Black (9% vs 12%) or Hispanic/Latinx (6% vs 10%).

Distribution of Outcomes of Interest

Tier 1 (nonsupervisors) and tier 2/3 (supervisors and executives) rural staff reported lower proficiency than urban staff in corresponding tiers in almost all skills; training needs aligned with responses indicating low proficiency. A lower proportion of rural than urban staff reported an intention to leave in the next year for reasons other than retirement (19% vs 25%, respectively). However, higher proportions of rural than urban staff reported an intent to leave because of COVID-19 (18% vs 15%), being bullied or harassed because of their work as public health professionals (22% vs 16%), and avoiding situations that made them think about COVID-19 (a PTSD symptom; 40% vs 36%).[1] Descriptive statistics regarding differences in rural versus urban responses to each skill, training need, intent to leave, and impact of COVID-19 are in Tables A and B (available as a supplement to the online version of this article at http://www.ajph.org).

Regression

Skills and training needs. Figure 1 presents logistic regression results on reported skill proficiencies. When we controlled for staff-, organizational-, and community-level factors, tier 1 rural staff, compared with urban staff, had significantly higher odds of reporting proficiency in 2 of 3 skill areas within the Community Engagement domain: "Describe the value of community strategic planning" (adjusted odds ratio [AOR] = 1.17; 95% confidence interval [CI] = 1.01, 1.35) and "Describe the importance of engaging community members in program design and implementation" (AOR = 1.17; 95% CI = 1.01, 1.35; skill names are abbreviated; full names are available in online Table C). Similarly, tier 1 rural staff had greater odds of reporting proficiency in the 2 skill areas specific to Cross-Sectoral Partnerships: "Collaborate with public health personnel across the agency" (AOR = 1.22; 95% CI = 1.05, 1.41) and "Engage community assets to improve health in a community" (AOR = 1.23; 95% CI = 1.07, 1.42). However, tier 1 rural staff had lower odds of reporting proficiency in the following skills: "Describe the value of a diverse workforce" (AOR = 0.84; 95% CI = 0.72, 0.99) and "Collect data for use in decision-making" (AOR = 0.83; 95% CI = 0.71, 0.99). Tier 1 rural staff skill deficiencies or proficiencies tended to be consistent with the presence or absence of training needs; specifically, in skill areas where rural staff were more likely than urban staff to report proficiencies (e.g., cross-sectoral partnerships), they were less likely to report training needs and vice versa with regard to areas where they were less likely to report proficiencies (e.g., data for use in decision-making; Figure 2).

In adjusted models, rural tier 2/3 staff had higher odds than urban staff of reporting proficiency in 7 of 24 skill areas (Figure 1). Similar to tier 1 rural staff, tier 2/3 rural staff had higher odds of reporting proficiency in 2 of 3 skill areas in the Community Engagement domains: "Engage community members in program design and implementation" (AOR = 1.27; 95% CI = 1.01, 1.60) and "Apply findings from a community health assessment" (AOR = 1.26; 95% CI = 1.00, 1.59). Tier 2/3 rural staff also had significantly higher odds of reporting skill proficiency in 3 of 4 areas related to Systems and Strategic Thinking: "Create a culture of/Apply quality improvement processes" (AOR = 1.30; 95% CI = 1.03, 1.64); "Implement/Ensure successful implementation of an organizational strategic plan" (AOR = 1.35; 95% CI = 1.09, 1.71); and "Build cross-sector partnerships to address social determinants of health" (AOR = 1.35; 95% CI = 1.08, 1.70). Furthermore, tier 2/3 staff were significantly less likely to have training needs in the latter 2 skill areas (AOR = 0.77 and 0.79, respectively;

TABLE 1— Selected Local Health Department (LHD) Personnel and Organizational Characteristics and Community Demographics, Stratified by Rural–Urban Designation: United States, 2021

	Total, No. (%) or Mean ±SD	Rural, No. (%) or Mean ±SD	Urban, No. (%) or Mean ±SD	P
		LHD Personnel		
Total sample	29 751 (100)	4 845 (16)	24 906 (84)	
Gender				< .001
Male	5 355 (18)	662 (14)	4 693 (19)	
Female	23 518 (79)	4 037 (83)	19 481 (79)	
Nonbinary/other	488 (2)	77 (2)	411 (2)	
Age, y				.1
< 31	3 877 (13)	588 (12)	3 289 (15)	
31–50	12 995 (44)	2 077 (43)	10 918 (44)	
≥ 50	9 936 (33)	1 708 (35)	8 228 (33)	
Race/ethnicity				< .001
American Indian or Alaska Native	276 (1)	69 (1)	207 (1)	
Asian	1 810 (6)	86 (2)	1 724 (7)	
Black or African American	4 327 (15)	306 (6)	4 021 (16)	
Hispanic or Latino	5 749 (19)	504 (10)	5 245 (21)	
Native Hawaiian or other Pacific Islander	95 (0.3)	9 (0.2)	86 (0.4)	
White	15 484 (52)	3 627 (75)	11 857 (48)	
≥ 2 races	1 238 (4)	132 (3)	1 106 (4)	
Supervisory status				.001
Nonsupervisor (tier 1)	22 316 (75)	3 704 (76)	18 612 (75)	
Supervisor/manager (tier 2)	6 700 (23)	1 003 (21)	5 697 (23)	
Executive (tier 3)	735 (2)	138 (3)	597 (2)	
Education level				< .001
Bachelor's degree or less	20 582 (69)	3 788 (78)	16 794 (67)	
Master's degree or higher	8 732 (29)	985 (20)	7 747 (31)	
Tenure in public health practice, y				.002
0–5	10 746 (36)	1 846 (38)	8 900 (36)	
≥ 5	17 376 (58)	2 711 (56)	14 665 (59)	
LHD organizational characteristics				
Lead executive is a clinician	10 812 (36)	1 058 (22)	9 754 (39)	< .001
Accredited	17 619 (59)	1 572 (32)	16 047 (64)	< .001
		Organizational Characteristics		
FTEs per 1000 population[a]	0.73 (1)	0.9 (1)	0.6 (1)	< .001
Community demographics				
Population, 1000s	238 (585)	33 (23)	410 (751)	< .001
Median household income, $1000s	59 (16)	51 (10)	65 (17)	< .001
% persons at or below federal poverty level[b]	14 (5)	15 (5)	12 (4)	< .001
% unemployed	3 (1)	3 (1)	3 (1)	< .001
% > 25 y with < high school diploma	8 (4)	9 (4)	7 (3)	< .001
% Black	11 (14)	9 (15)	12 (13)	< .001

Continued

TABLE 1— Continued

	Total, No. (%) or Mean ±SD	Rural, No. (%) or Mean ±SD	Urban, No. (%) or Mean ±SD	P
% American Indian/Alaska Native	2 (5)	3 (6)	1 (3)	<.001
% Hispanic/Latinx	8 (10)	6 (8)	10 (12)	<.001

Note. FTE = full-time equivalent employee; LHD = local health department.

[a]This was calculated using LHD FTEs reported in the 2019 National Association of City and County Health Officials Profile of Local Health Departments survey and the 2020 population for that area (FTEs/population × 1000).
[b]According to US Census criteria.

Figure 2). Skill proficiencies and training needs were also aligned in the Data-Based Decision-Making domain: rural tier 2/3 staff had significantly lower odds of reporting proficiency in "Use valid data" (AOR = 0.70; 95% CI = 0.53, 0.93) and significantly higher odds of having a training need in this area (AOR = 1.46; 95% CI = 1.10, 1.55).

Turnover risk and COVID-19 impact. In logistic regression analyses of turnover risk and impact of COVID-19 (Figure 3), rural staff across all tiers were less likely than urban staff to report an intent to leave in the next year (AOR = 0.73; 95% CI = 0.64, 0.83). They were also less likely to report an intent to leave because of lack of acknowledgment or recognition (AOR = 0.73), lack of opportunities for advancement (AOR = 0.69), pay (AOR = 0.67), and lack of flexibility (AOR = 0.51). However, when we restricted the sample to staff intending to leave in the next year (excluding retirements, n = 7185), the odds of rural staff reporting an intent to leave because of stress were higher than those of urban staff (AOR = 1.29; 95% CI = 1.02, 1.60; results not shown); other relationships were unchanged in this analysis. The odds of rural participants reporting that they had been bullied or harassed because of their work were 1.22 times the odds for urban staff (95% CI = 1.04, 1.32). In addition, rural staff had higher odds than urban staff of reporting that they avoided situations that made them think about COVID-19 (AOR = 1.15; 95% CI = 1.04, 1.27).

DISCUSSION

Our findings provide novel information regarding rural–urban differences in skills, training needs, turnover risks, and the impact of COVID-19 on the workforce. They also suggest areas of rural strength and concern. We found that compared with urban LHD staff, rural LHD staff reported greater proficiency in skills related to community engagement, cross-sectoral partnerships, and systems thinking, but had greater training needs in areas related to data-based decision-making and to justice, equity, diversity, and inclusion. We also found that rural LHD staff were more likely than urban staff to report being harassed by individuals outside of their LHD because of their work. Despite harassment, rural staff were less likely than urban staff to report an intent to leave their organization. However, of staff reporting intentions to leave, rural participants were more likely to report stress as a reason for leaving; rural staff were also more likely to report avoiding situations reminding them of COVID-19, which is a PTSD symptom.

The rural–urban differences we identified highlight opportunities for public health workforce development. Rural staff proficiencies in community engagement, cross-sectoral partnerships, and systems and strategic thinking skills are important for accomplishing public health work—especially in rural communities[3]—providing an opportunity to build on these rural assets during staff trainings and offering lessons for urban LHDs. In addition, research examining general public health workforce capacity during and before the pandemic found training needs with regard to connecting effectively with populations that have negative perceptions of public health; our findings suggest that rural staff may be good resources in developing such training.[28] Finally, previous research indicates that LHD directors with nursing backgrounds are skilled in communication, collaboration, and partnering with communities.[14,26] Because many rural LHDs are led and staffed by nurses, our findings may reflect the presence of nurses and suggest the efficacy of nursing leadership, which has been found by others.[14,26]

At the same time, skill gaps among rural staff, such as those related to data-based decision-making and to justice, equity, diversity, and inclusion, point to priorities for focusing rural

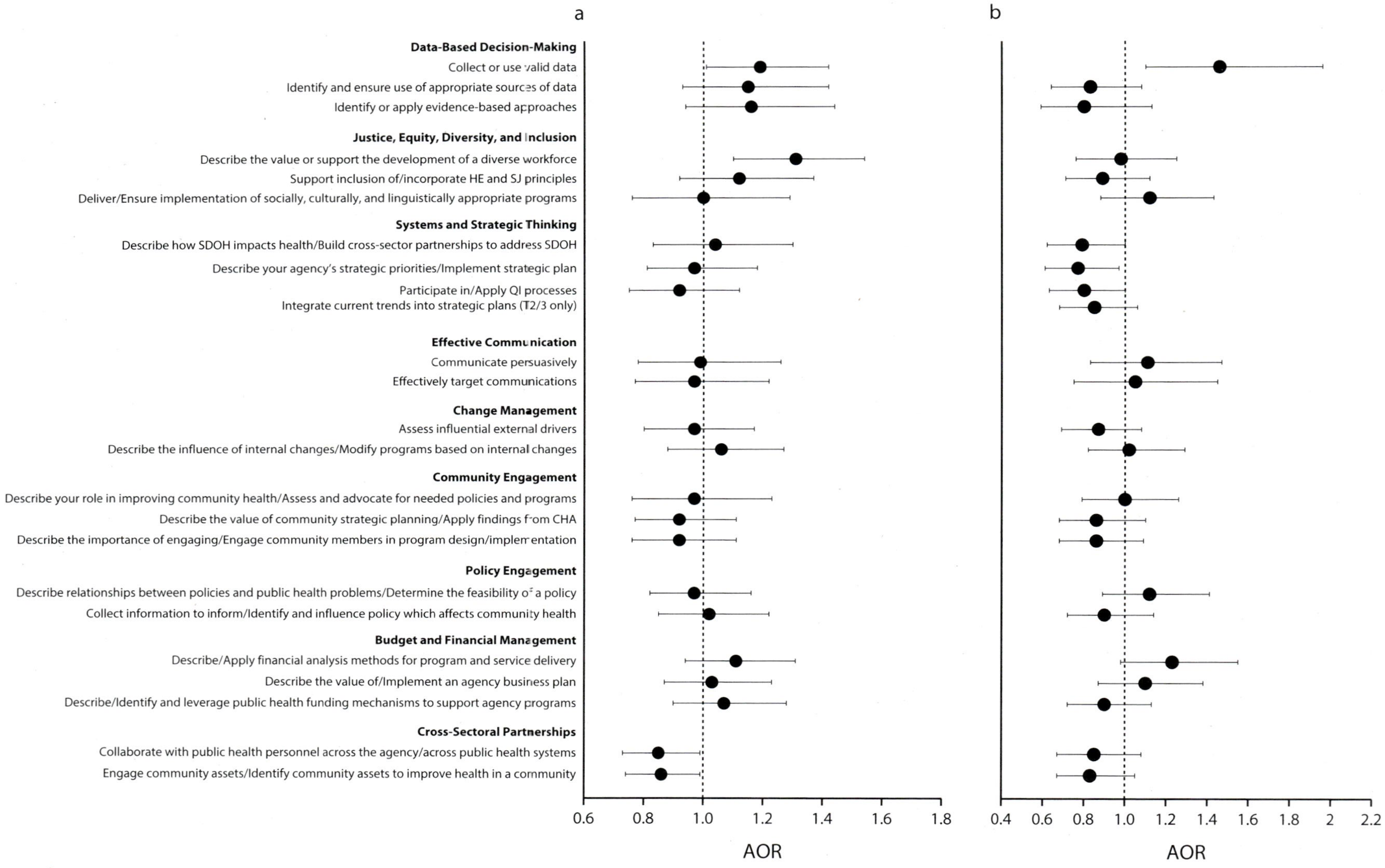

FIGURE 2— **Rural vs Urban Training Needs Among Nonsupervisors and Supervisors/Executives in Local Health Departments by (a) Tier 1 Training Needs and (b) Tier 2/3 Training Needs: United States, 2021**

Note. AOR = adjusted odds ratio; CHA = community health assessment; HE = health equity; QI = quality improvement; SDOH = social determinants of health; SJ = social justice. All results of the logistic regression are presented in their exponentiated form as odds ratios with urban as the reference category; AOR = 1.0 is not statistically significant. All outcomes are adjusted for local health department organizational variables (clinician-led, accreditation, full-time equivalent employees per 1000 population), staff variables (tenure, education level), and community-level variables (% unemployed, % in poverty, % older than 25 years with < high school diploma, % Black population, % Hispanic population, and % American Indian/Alaska Native population). Numerical values are available in Table C (available as a supplement to the online version of this article at http://www.ajph.org). Skill names are abbreviated; full names are available in online Table C. Skills with a "/" indicate tier 1 and tier 2/3 wording; tier 2/3 wording follows the "/".

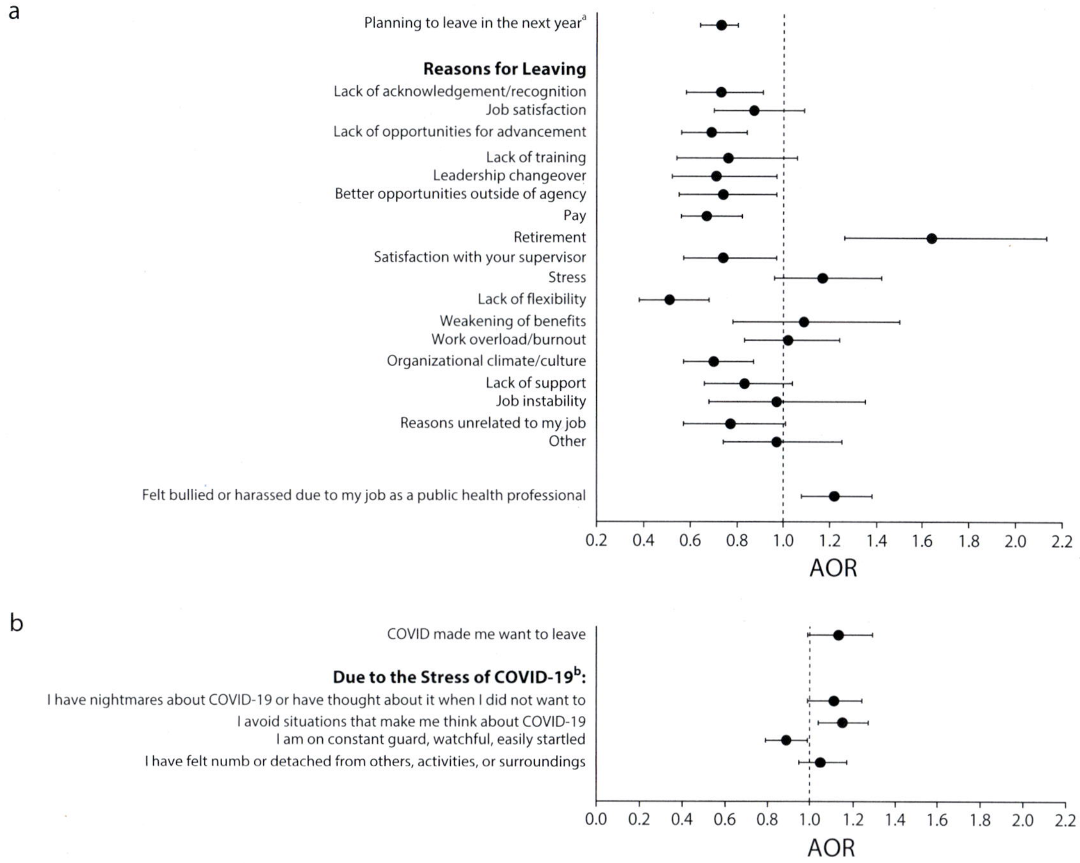

FIGURE 3— Regression Results Among Local Health Department Nonsupervisors, Supervisors, and Executives of (a) Rural vs Urban Intention to Leave and (b) Impact of COVID-19: United States, 2021

Note. AOR = adjusted odds ratio. All results are presented in their exponential form as AORs with urban as the reference category; AOR = 1.0 is not statistically significant. All outcomes are adjusted for local health department organizational variables (clinician-led, accreditation, full-time equivalent employees per 1000 population), staff variables (tenure, education level), and community-level variables (% unemployed, % in poverty, % older than 25 years with < high school diploma, % Black population, % Hispanic population, and % American Indian/Alaska Native population). Numerical values of AORs and confidence intervals can be found in Table D (available as a supplement to the online version of this article at http://www.ajph.org). Results are presented at the total staff level (nonsupervisors, supervisors, and executives) rather than by staff tiers.

[a]Excludes retirement.

[b]PTSD screening tool. The lead-in for this question was: "Has the coronavirus or COVID-19 outbreak been so frightening, horrible, or unsettling that . . . ."

workforce development efforts. With respect to skill gaps in justice, equity, diversity, and inclusion, some rural communities have previously been predominantly White and relatively homogenous, but increasing rural diversity may be prompting rural staffs' recognition of the need for these skills. The lack of diversity among rural staff themselves may also be contributing to, and prompting, this training need.[3,15,29] Collectively, gaps in both data-based decision-making and justice, equity, diversity, and inclusion may have affected rural LHD staff's preparedness for COVID-19 and contributed to their stress, because data collection and analysis as well as abilities to address diverse community needs were important skills needed during the pandemic.[12,30,31] Given that rates of COVID-19 infections were high in rural areas, findings suggest that resources should be allocated to address known skill gaps, such as use of data in decision-making, and support growth of a more diverse workforce to enable rural staff to effectively serve marginalized members of increasingly diverse rural communities.[30,32,33]

Our findings also show that COVID-19 significantly affected rural staff, compounding prepandemic stressors from underfunding and inadequate workforce capacity.[34] Along with greater odds of reporting skill gaps in areas essential for COVID-19 responsiveness, proportionally more rural staff reported wanting to leave because of COVID-19 and overload or burnout. Further, burnout and stress were the second and third most common reasons rural LHD staff listed for wanting to leave. This is in contrast to state and large- or medium-sized health department respondents in the 2017 PH WINS national sample survey, where the second and third most common reasons for wanting to leave were lack of opportunities for advancement and workplace environment.[20] Our study highlights the impact of stress and COVID-19 on rural LHD staff as evidenced by their greater odds of wanting to leave because of stress, of avoiding situations that made them think about COVID-19, and of experiencing bullying or harassment. At the same time, even as they appear to have suffered greater stress and harassment than urban counterparts, rural staff had less intention to leave their job soon. Rural staffs' reasons for intending to remain in their positions, despite notable challenges, deserve further investigation.

Limitations

Our cross-sectional design limits the ability to determine causality. We also lack data on numbers of staff that have left their jobs, limiting a comprehensive understanding of the pandemic's impact and how turnover risk translates to actual turnover. Furthermore, skill proficiencies and training needs may look different if formally assessed rather than self-reported. Finally, the inability to incorporate weights because of our inclusion of small LHDs in Regions 5 and 10 may affect generalizability. Despite these limitations, evidence here regarding rural public health workers can inform important future workforce research.

Public Health Implications

Rural LHD staff face multiple pressures and changes to practice while grappling with the long-term impacts of COVID-19 and increasing diversity in their communities. Rural staff have also been challenged both to provide clinical services and to increase their focus on population-based services while responding to a pandemic. They do this work with limited resources, including inadequate funds and staffing.[8,15] Our findings offer novel evidence regarding rural staff skills and training gaps, providing evidence for effectively supporting and strengthening this workforce to ensure readiness for future emergencies. Greater investment is needed in rural public health workforce development that is based on the assets and needs of rural staff and rural communities, including areas related to data collection and use.[16,35] Opportunities also exist to leverage rural staff competencies in systems thinking and community partnership for the lessons they can offer urban LHD staff. Finally, this study highlights urgent needs to address turnover risk and reported stress, burnout, and experiences of bullying and harassment that have taken place during the pandemic, especially for rural staff. Ensuring a resilient, prepared, and thriving rural workforce is critical to equitably addressing community health needs and responding to future pandemics. AJPH

ABOUT THE AUTHORS

Paula M. Kett and Davis G. Patterson are with the Center for Health Workforce Studies, Department of Family Medicine, and Betty Bekemeier is with the School of Nursing, University of Washington, Seattle. Kay Schaffer is with the de Beaumont Foundation, Bethesda, MD.

CORRESPONDENCE

Correspondence should be sent to Paula M. Kett, PhD, MPH, RN, UW Center for Health Workforce Studies, Department of Family Medicine, University of Washington, Box 354982, Seattle, WA 98195-4982 (e-mail: pmk@uw.edu). Reprints can be ordered at http://www.ajph.org by clicking the "Reprints" link.

PUBLICATION INFORMATION

Full Citation: Kett PM, Bekemeier B, Patterson DG, Schaffer K. Competencies, training needs, and turnover among rural compared with urban local public health practitioners: 2021 Public Health Workforce Interests and Needs Survey. *Am J Public Health*. 2023;113(6):689–699.

Acceptance Date: February 19, 2023.

DOI: https://doi.org/10.2105/AJPH.2023.307273

CONTRIBUTORS

P. M. Kett conceptualized and provided the first draft of this article, with contributions from B. Bekemeier, D. G. Patterson, and K. Schaffer. All authors contributed to editing and revising the article and approved the final version.

ACKNOWLEDGMENTS

This study was supported by the Health Resources and Services Administration (HRSA) of the US Department of Health and Human Services (HHS) as part of an award totaling $536 449 with zero percentage financed with nongovernmental sources. Data for this study were obtained from the Public Health Workforce Interests and Needs Survey, a project supported through a collaboration of the Association of State and Territorial Health Officials (ASTHO) and the de Beaumont Foundation.

Note. The contents are those of the authors and do not necessarily represent the official views of, nor an endorsement by, the HRSA, HHS, or the US Government. For more information, please visit HRSA.gov. The use of the data does not imply ASTHO or the de Beaumont Foundation's endorsement of the research, research methods, or conclusions contained in this report.

CONFLICTS OF INTEREST

There are no conflicts of interest to disclose.

HUMAN PARTICIPANT PROTECTION

The University of Washington institutional review board deemed this study exempt.

REFERENCES

1. de Beaumont Foundation and Association of State and Territorial Health Officials. Public Health Workforce Interest and Needs Survey: 2021 findings. 2022. Available at: https://debeaumont.org/phwins/2021-findings. Accessed September 6, 2022.

2. Smith MR, Weber L. Health officials are quitting or getting fired amid outbreak. *Associated Press.* August 10, 2020. Available at: https://apnews.com/article/virus-outbreak-u-s-news-ap-top-news-ok-state-wire-ca-state-wire-8ea3b3669bccf8a637b81f8261f1cd78. Accessed September 6, 2022.
3. Grimm B, Ramos AK, Maloney S, et al. The most important skills required by local public health departments for responding to community needs and improving health outcomes. *J Community Health.* 2022;47(1):79–86. https://doi.org/10.1007/s10900-021-01020-0
4. Robin N, Castrucci BC, McGinty MD, Edmiston A, Bogaert K. The first nationally representative benchmark of the local governmental public health workforce: findings from the 2017 Public Health Workforce Interests and Needs Survey. *J Public Health Manag Pract.* 2019;25(suppl 2):S26–S37. https://doi.org/10.1097/PHH.0000000000000939
5. Beck AJ, Leider JP, Coronado F, Harper E. State health agency and local health department workforce: identifying top development needs. *Am J Public Health.* 2017;107(9):1418–1424. https://doi.org/10.2105/AJPH.2017.303875
6. Leider JP, Meit M, McCullough JM, et al. The state of rural public health: enduring needs in a new decade. *Am J Public Health.* 2020;110(9):1283–1290. https://doi.org/10.2105/AJPH.2020.305728
7. Bekemeier B, Park S, Backonja U, Ornelas I, Turner AM. Data, capacity-building, and training needs to address rural health inequities in the Northwest United States: a qualitative study. *J Am Med Inform Assoc.* 2019;26(8–9):825–834. https://doi.org/10.1093/jamia/ocz037
8. Leider J, Henning-Smith C. Resourcing public health to meet the needs of rural America. *Am J Public Health.* 2020;110(9):1291–1292. https://doi.org/10.2105/AJPH.2020.305818
9. DeSalvo K, Wang Y, Harris A, Auerbach J, Koo D, O'Carroll P. Public health 3.0: a call to action for public health to meet the challenges of the 21st century. *Prev Chronic Dis.* 2017;14:170017. https://doi.org/10.5888/pcd14.170017
10. Stamatakis KA, Baker EA, McVay A, Keedy H. Development of a measurement tool to assess local public health implementation climate and capacity for equity-oriented practice: application to obesity prevention in a local public health system. *PLoS One.* 2020;15(9):e0237380. https://doi.org/10.1371/journal.pone.0237380
11. National Academy of Medicine. *Emerging Stronger From COVID-19: Priorities for Health System Transformation.* Washington, DC: National Academies Press; 2022. https://doi.org/10.17226/26657
12. Brownson RC, Burke TA, Colditz GA, Samet JM. Reimagining public health in the aftermath of a pandemic. *Am J Public Health.* 2020;110(11):1605–1610. https://doi.org/10.2105/AJPH.2020.305861
13. Hogg-Graham R, Graves E, Mays GP. Identifying value-added population health capabilities to strengthen public health infrastructure. *Milbank Q.* 2022;100(1):261–283. https://doi.org/10.1111/1468-0009.12553
14. *2019 National Profile of Local Health Departments.* Washington, DC: National Association of County and City Health Officials; 2020.
15. Harris JK, Beatty K, Leider JP, Knudson A, Anderson AJ, Meit M. The double disparity facing rural local health departments. *Annu Rev Public Health.* 2016;37(1):167–184. https://doi.org/10.1146/annurev-publhealth-031914-122755
16. Sainkhuu S, Cunha-Cruz J, Knerr S, Rogers M, Bekemeier B. Evaluation of training gaps among public health practitioners in Washington State. *J Public Health Manag Pract.* 2021;27(5):473–483. https://doi.org/10.1097/PHH.0000000000001184
17. Leider JP, Sellers K, Owens-Young J, et al. Determinants of workplace perceptions among federal, state, and local public health staff in the US, 2014 to 2017. *BMC Public Health.* 2021;21(1):1654. https://doi.org/10.1186/s12889-021-11703-x
18. McFarlane TD, Dixon BE, Grannis SJ, Gibson PJ. Public health informatics in local and state health agencies: an update from the public health workforce interests and needs survey. *J Public Health Manag Pract.* 2019;25(suppl 2):S67–S77. https://doi.org/10.1097/PHH.0000000000000918
19. Yeager VA, Balio CP, Kronstadt J, Beitsch LM. The relationship between health department accreditation and workforce satisfaction, retention, and training needs. *J Public Health Manag Pract.* 2019;25(suppl 2):S113–S123. https://doi.org/10.1097/PHH.0000000000000920
20. Bogaert K, Castrucci BC, Gould E, et al. The Public Health Workforce Interests and Needs Survey (PH WINS 2017): an expanded perspective on the state health agency workforce. *J Public Health Manag Pract.* 2019;25(suppl 2):S16–S25. https://doi.org/10.1097/PHH.0000000000000932
21. Harper E, Castrucci BC, Bharthapudi K, Sellers K. Job satisfaction: a critical, understudied facet of workforce development in public health. *J Public Health Manag Pract.* 2015;21(suppl 6):S46–S55. https://doi.org/10.1097/PHH.0000000000000296
22. Sellers K, Leider JP, Bogaert K, Allen JD, Castrucci BC. Making a living in governmental public health: variation in earnings by employee characteristics and work setting. *J Public Health Manag Pract.* 2019;25(suppl 2):S87–S95. https://doi.org/10.1097/PHH.0000000000000935
23. Taylor HL, Yeager VA. Core competency gaps among governmental public health employees with and without a formal public health degree. *J Public Health Manag Pract.* 2021;27(1):20–29. https://doi.org/10.1097/PHH.0000000000001071
24. Kulik P, Leider JP, Rogers R, et al. PH WINS for all: the critical role of partnerships for engaging all local health departments in the Public Health Workforce Interest and Needs Survey. *J Public Health Manag Pract.* 2023;29(suppl 1):S48–S53. https://doi.org/10.1097/PHH.0000000000001635
25. Bekemeier B, Grembowski D, Yang Y, Herting JR. Leadership matters: local health department clinician leaders and their relationship to decreasing health disparities. *J Public Health Manag Pract.* 2012;18(2):E1–E10. https://doi.org/10.1097/PHH.0b013e318242d4fc
26. Kett PM, Bekemeier B, Herting JR, Altman MR. Addressing health disparities: the health department nurse lead executive's relationship to improved community health. *J Public Health Manag Pract.* 2022;28(2):E566–E576. https://doi.org/10.1097/PHH.0000000000001425
27. Robins M, Leider J, Schaffer K, Gambatese M, Allen E, Hare Bork R. WINS 2021 Methodology Report. *J Public Health Manag Pract.* 2023; 29(suppl 1):S35–S44. https://doi.org/10.1097/PHH.0000000000001632
28. Zemmel DJ, Kulik PKG, Leider JP, Power LE. Public health workforce development during and beyond the COVID-19 pandemic: findings from a qualitative training needs assessment. *J Public Health Manag Pract.* 2022;28(suppl 5):S263–S270. https://doi.org/10.1097/PHH.0000000000001524
29. Rowlands D, Love H. Mapping rural America's diversity and demographic change. *The Avenue.* 2021. Available at: https://www.brookings.edu/blog/the-avenue/2021/09/28/mapping-rural-americas-diversity-and-demographic-change. Accessed August 24, 2022.
30. Czabanowska K, Kuhlmann E. Public health competences through the lens of the COVID-19 pandemic: what matters for health workforce preparedness for global health emergencies. *Int J Health Plann Manage.* 2021;36(S1):14–19. https://doi.org/10.1002/hpm.3131
31. Callaghan T, Lueck JA, Trujillo KL, Ferdinand AO. Rural and urban differences in COVID-19 prevention behaviors. *J Rural Health.* 2021;37(2):287–295. https://doi.org/10.1111/jrh.12556
32. Dearinger AT. COVID-19 reveals emerging opportunities for rural public health. *Am J Public Health.* 2020;110(9):1277–1278. https://doi.org/10.2105/AJPH.2020.305864
33. Dobis EA, McGranahan D. Rural residents appear to be more vulnerable to serious infection or death from COVID-19. *Amber Waves.* US Dept of Agriculture, Economic Research Service. 2021. Available at: https://www.ers.usda.gov/amber-waves/2021/february/rural-residents-appear-to-be-more-vulnerable-to-serious-infection-or-death-from-coronavirus-covid-19. Accessed on January 26, 2023.
34. Melvin SC, Wiggins C, Burse N, Thompson E, Monger M. The role of public health in COVID-19 emergency response efforts from a rural health perspective. *Prev Chronic Dis.* 2020;17:200256. https://doi.org/10.5888/pcd17.200256
35. Backonja U, Park S, Kurre A, et al. Supporting rural public health practice to address local-level social determinants of health across Northwest states: development of an interactive visualization dashboard. *J Biomed Inform.* 2022;129:104051. https://doi.org/10.1016/j.jbi.2022.104051

7

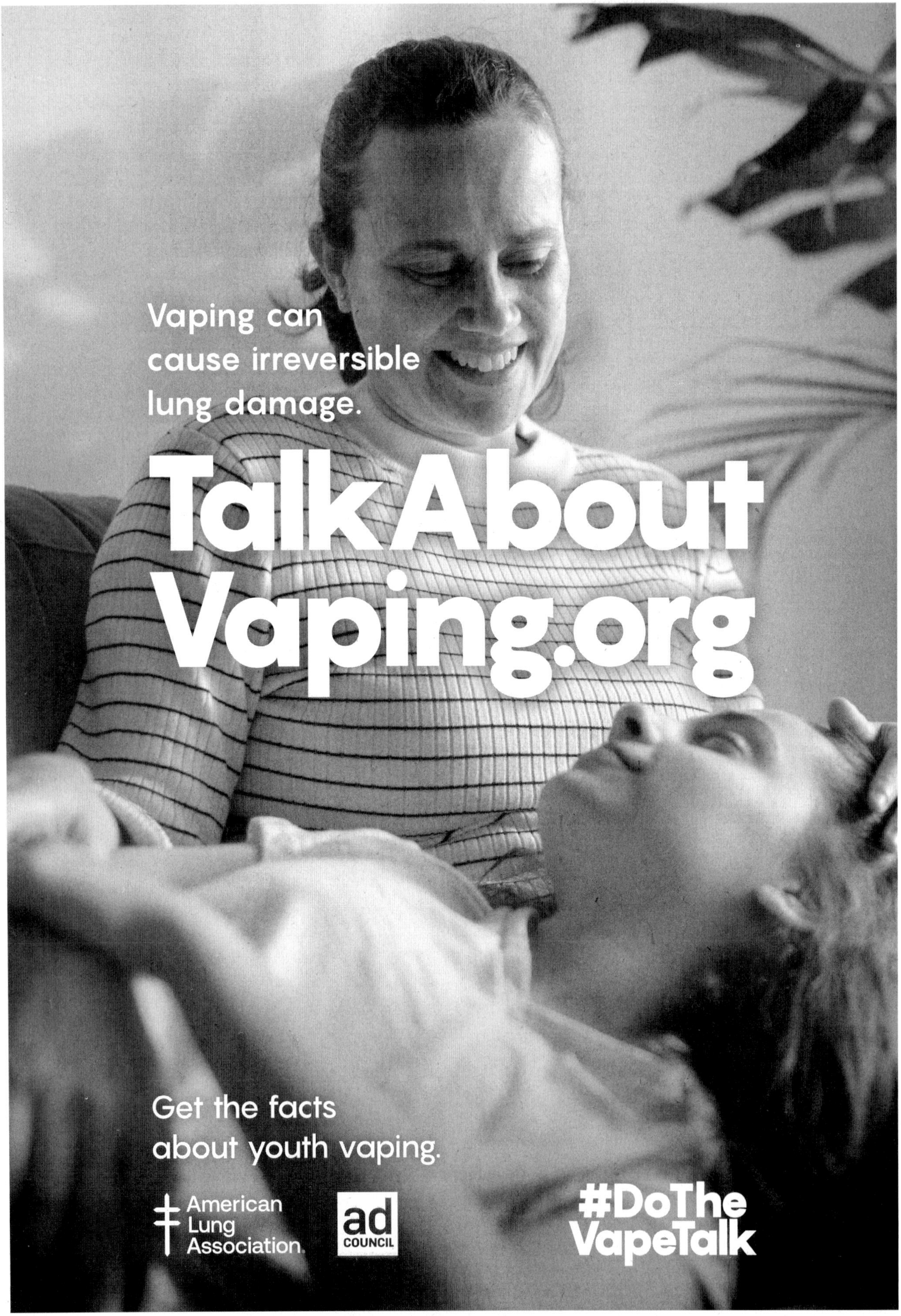
Vaping can
cause irreversible
lung damage.
TalkAbout
Vaping.org
Get the facts
about youth vaping.
American
Lung
Association.
ad
COUNCIL
#DoThe
VapeTalk

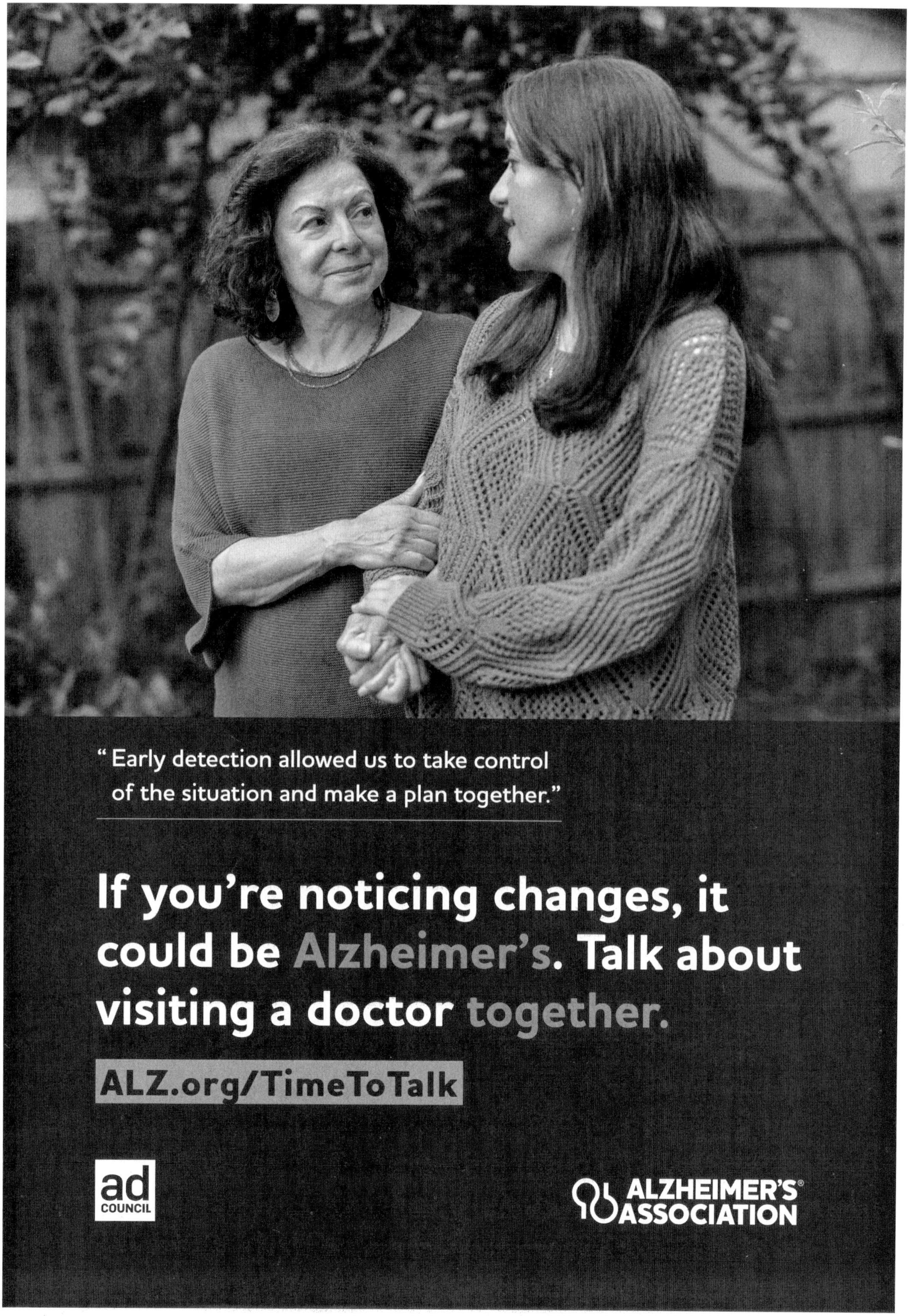
" Early detection allowed us to take control of the situation and make a plan together."
If you're noticing changes, it could be Alzheimer's. Talk about visiting a doctor together.
ALZ.org/TimeToTalk
ad COUNCIL
ALZHEIMER'S® ASSOCIATION

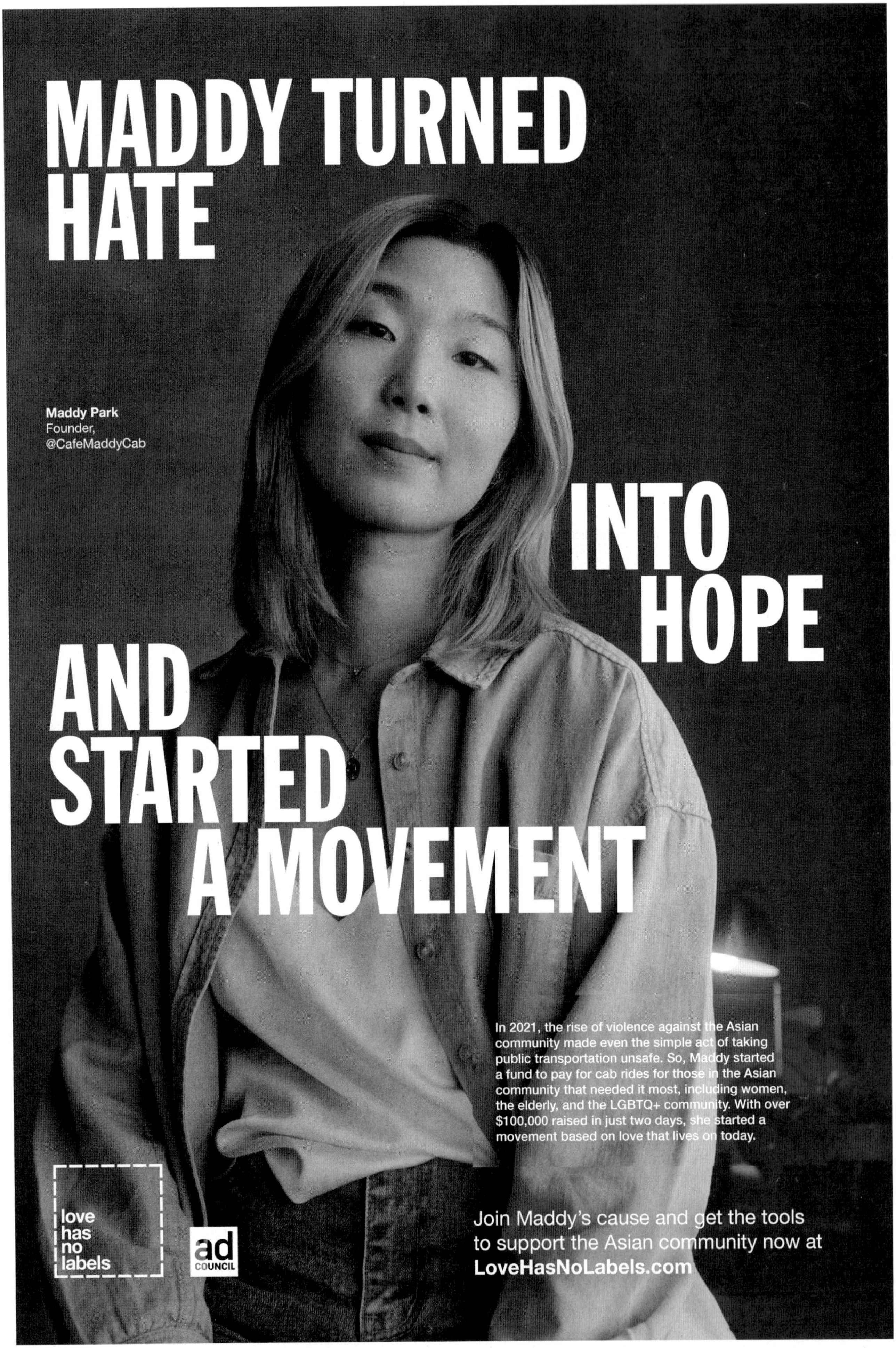

MADDY TURNED HATE
INTO HOPE
AND STARTED A MOVEMENT
Maddy Park
Founder,
@CafeMaddyCab
In 2021, the rise of violence against the Asian community made even the simple act of taking public transportation unsafe. So, Maddy started a fund to pay for cab rides for those in the Asian community that needed it most, including women, the elderly, and the LGBTQ+ community. With over $100,000 raised in just two days, she started a movement based on love that lives on today.
love has no labels
ad COUNCIL
Join Maddy's cause and get the tools to support the Asian community now at
LoveHasNoLabels.com

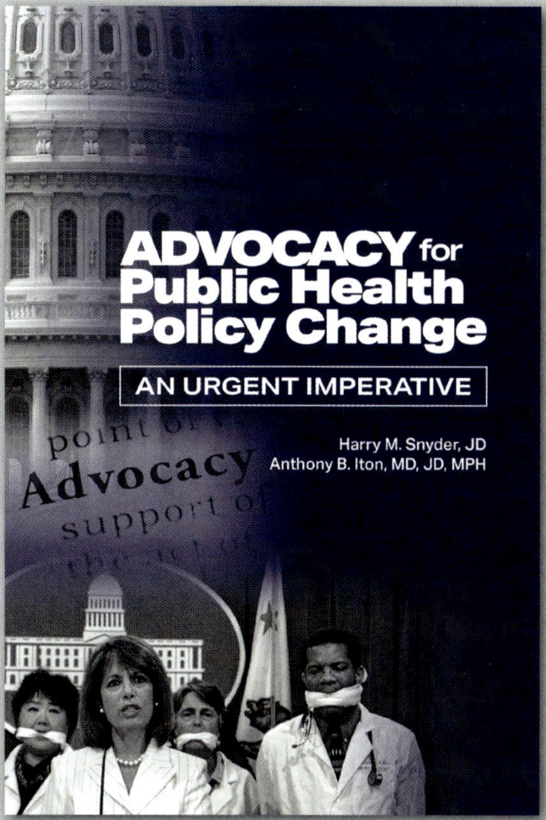

Advocacy for Public Health Policy Change: An Urgent Imperative

Edited by Harry M. Snyder, MD
Anthony B. Iton, MD, JD, MPH

Improving laws and policies start with advocacy and now more than ever this new book, *Advocacy for Public Health Policy Change: An Urgent Imperative* will be instrumental in training public health practitioners and students to turn their expertise into sound policies and laws. It will help these readers in these five key areas:

- Address the growing need to turn knowledge into better health policy.
- Offer a step-by-step planning and implementation framework for public health advocacy campaigns from start to finish.
- Expand professional development and satisfactions opportunities for the field.
- Improve service delivery.
- Improve health outcomes.

Place orders at **aphabookstore.org**. Email **bookstoreservices@apha.org** to request an exam copy for classroom use.

ISBN 978-0-87553-313-1 2020, SOFTCOVER, 250 PAGES

APHA PRESS
AN IMPRINT OF **AMERICAN PUBLIC HEALTH ASSOCIATION**